Whistle in the Wind

PETER DUFFY FRCS MD

Peter's love for his family and for what he does as a surgeon runs through the pages of this gripping book as he takes you on a journey to some of the darker areas of our NHS and legal system. As a society we need to face up to the appalling reality of what the NHS does to staff that speak up and how much public money it wastes fighting people that act in the public interest. Even a committed, award winning surgeon who transformed cancer services was not immune from attempts by the NHS to destroy him when he decided to stand up for patients and services. This is everyone's problem.

Dr Chris Day, junior doctor and whistle-blower

Peter's book should be compulsory reading for all medical undergraduates. It should also be read by individuals who work for the BMA, GMC and CQC. We should be grateful that a courageous doctor like Peter is out there. He serves to remind the rest of us of what we are here for.

Senior consultant, Noble's Hospital

An absorbing and sometimes disturbing story of an NHS whistle-blower.

Consultant surgeon and ex-colleague, NHS England

A very readable account of a consultant surgeon's disturbing experience of the costs of whistleblowing. Essential reading for all in Senior Management positions in the NHS.

Senior GP, Lancaster

I had a colleague with whom I could discuss complicated patients and ask his opinion, assist with complex operations and regard as a friend. Peter's relationship with staff and patients was exceptionally good. I am stopped in the street by former patients who wish him well and would love to see him back.

Mr Richard Wilson FRCS, consultant urological surgeon, NHS England

This is a chilling indictment of how the modern NHS now operates, and the Orwellian nightmare it has become. I have the utmost respect for those willing to stand up and be counted, but most of us remain too afraid to do so.

Anon

Senior consultant, Noble's Hospital

While much tremendous work is carried out by the NHS on a daily basis, ...when things do go wrong, there is a huge failure in acknowledging mistakes and more importantly learning from them.

In my case at the Trust Peter refers to, despite many scans and consultations over three years my cancer was not correctly diagnosed until another Trust carried out an unrelated scan. The first Trust continued to tell me everything was alright but after proving this was incorrect, I attempted to find out how so many mistakes could be made... and whether other patients were similarly impacted.

What followed over almost two years were cover ups, delays, evasions, failures to produce critical documents and deliberate misinformation from the medical team right up to the highest levels of Trust management. In July 2019 I am still fighting to get a proper review of my case!

Current NHS urological surgery patient

Dedicated to the values, commitment, professionalism and hard work of two of my most loved and valued mentors:-

Mr Bob Thomson FRCS
Consultant urological surgeon

Mr Richard Wilson FRCS
Consultant urological surgeon

"To err is human, to cover up is unforgivable and to fail to learn is inexcusable"

Professor Sir Liam Donaldson
Former Chief Medical Officer, England

Foreword

I WILL ALWAYS ADMIRE the fortitude and commitment of professionals such as Peter, who speak up to protect others, at great personal cost to themselves. I have been able to provide some support to Peter throughout his difficult journey, but by no means the amount that he and other whistle-blowers need and deserve. Sadly, there is much need to improve the experience of whistle-blowers in health and other sectors. Not least to ensure that individuals are properly protected from the very outset, before harm is done. While some clear in roads have been made in more recent years, the reality is that experience is still inconsistent for individuals when they raise concerns internally. We know that many whistle-blowers prevail, they are not harmed, and patients are thereby protected. However, many whistle-blowers are ignored or victimised regardless of how clear, reasonable and consistent they have been. This is inexcusable in any organisation, let alone one whose primary purpose is healthcare. Furthermore, Peter's experience of litigation is one that is far too common for many whistle-blowers, where the balance of power is incredibly difficult and the ability to present your own case and evidence substantially hampered and outgunned.

We know of good work happening in the NHS, even though this did not benefit Peter. We hope that this will begin to address the inconsistencies we see in practice, by organisations learning from each other when they fail or succeed. However, individuals and organisations must be held to account when they fall short of standards and these standards must be clearly set by Government and other public bodies. In our 25 year history I have still only heard of one case where an individual was disciplined for victimising a whistle-blower, yet we hear from thousands of individuals who say they are suffering because they spoke up. This is a problem that all of society should see as their issue; we must protect those who speak up to protect us.

I hope that in telling his story it will highlight the much-needed reform of the law and the problems whistle-blowers face in accessing justice. More importantly I hope it will give some comfort to the public to know that there are so many dedicated professionals working in our beloved NHS that will speak up to protect patients, but also demonstrate how vitally important it is that when whistle-blowers speak up, they are heard and protected.

Francesca West
Chief Executive
Protect (formerly Public Concern at Work)
The Green House,
244-254 Cambridge Heath Rd,
London,
E2 9DA

Prologue

I'VE NEVER WRITTEN A BOOK BEFORE. I almost certainly never will again. This manuscript is forged out of a determination to get my story told whatever the barriers, threats and obstacles put in my way. There is no fiction or exaggeration. This is how it is, was and is likely to continue to be. The cold, brutal reality of low standards, poor behaviour, *laissez-faire* and cover-ups that seem to be an integral part of some contemporary NHS hospital, medical and surgical practice.

My vocation and training are relatively uncontroversial. My life as a consultant surgeon is not. This account of my years of service to the populations of North Lancashire and Cumbria and my response to the allegations and accusations levelled at me will undoubtedly be both disputed and subject to forensic legal examination. As such, I have had to draw heavily upon my witness statement and evidence presented to the Manchester Employment Tribunal. The material upon which this book is based is true, structured to withstand hostile cross-examination, founded on written evidence and exhaustively cross-referenced to the legal bundle.

Exposing dangerous practice and cover-ups at the highest level in the NHS, my story reveals issues which have the potential to seriously affect public safety. As a consequence, I strongly believe that it is in the public interest that my full story is told. If this book contributes to the safeguarding of some of society's most vulnerable individuals then the time spent putting this story together will not have been wasted.

In addition, I believe my reputation to have been wrongfully smeared with public accusations of racism and fraud made against me. This book is an opportunity for me to set the record straight, something that can only be done by telling the full story.

Based in sections upon my witness statement, legal submissions and medical statements presented to the Employment Tribunal, in parts my account will appear laboured, but bear with me. It is an evidence validated story of NHS risk taking and lax standards, cover-ups, lies, hypocrisy, abuse, deceit and corruption that is, I believe, well worthy of the telling.

I have restricted the opening chapters to no more than is necessary; introducing myself, my vocation, training and family. Deliberately keeping the introduction to well under 20% of the book as a whole, I hope that this will nevertheless inform the reader of who I am and of my early life choices.

The substantive section of Part I deals with my life as a consultant surgeon, working for the University Hospitals of Morecambe Bay NHS Foundation Trust in North West England. It details my legitimate and escalating clinical concerns and whistle-blowing, closely followed by my illegal constructive dismissal. Part II deals with the aftermath of my dismissal and the legal process that followed.

This is not a memoir or autobiography. It skims over or ignores issues that are not immediately relevant to public safety, clinical standards and whistle-blower protection. It quotes widely from evidentially important emails, conversations and the witness statement. As a consequence, is heavy in legal and particularly medical detail which I will do my best to explain as we go along.

Patient details and the details of staff who are not immediately relevant to the story are, of course, concealed.

Acknowledgements

First and foremost must be my family. Fiona, Edward, Robert and William have been utterly steadfast in their support, never once questioning whether the cost of my actions to them as well as to me has been worth it. My extended family too, have been robust and entirely supportive of the position that I have taken on clinical standards.

Old school friends Michael, David, Andrew and Mark have kept in touch and supported me through the darker times of the last two to three years, as well as some of my old colleagues and managers who for their own sake ought to remain nameless. Michael's advice in particular was invaluable and I'm very, very grateful to him for the many hours that he spent, reading through documents and statements.

The BMA came good with support when I was most in need of it. I am very grateful to them and I remain indebted to Chris Thompson and Paras Gorasia, my solicitor and barrister for their expert management of my case.

Francesca West, Chief Executive of Public Concern at Work (now *Protect*, the whistle-blowing charity) was invaluable and gave up much of her time including precious family evenings, to support me through the dark days and nights of the Tribunal process.

Dr Alison Birtle, consultant clinical oncologist and the only close colleague who stepped forward and was prepared to be a witness for me.

Drs' Chris Till and Dave Highley, for throwing me a career life line when I most needed it.

The staff at Noble's Hospital, Isle of Man and particularly my new urology colleagues Steve, Jackie, Julie, Marie and Emily, who have helped restore my faith in and enjoyment of clinical practice.

Nicola Thatcher, consultant solicitor for her professional support and expert advice.

Lastly, my family again. Not a day goes past when I don't dream of being back home and reunited with them.

Contents

Introduction

OUR NATIONAL HEALTH SERVICE is a truly great institution, perhaps the single greatest achievement of post-war Britain. Over the decades, innumerable lives have been prolonged by the millions of selfless, committed and largely un-thanked individuals who have devoted their entire working lives to the NHS. The NHS is the largest employer in Western Europe and we regularly hold it up as being one of the finest examples of socialised, free-at-the-point-of-delivery healthcare in the entire world. Looking back to the truly shocking healthcare conditions endured by our grandparents and those before them, it is impossible not to be grateful to this great organisation and all that its employees have done to eradicate some of the terrible plagues of recent times.

Tuberculosis, polio, syphilis, diphtheria, smallpox and more are now all but gone or entirely eradicated from the UK as a result of the labours of the NHS. People no longer routinely die in childbirth or from easily treated conditions like pneumonia or appendicitis. In the event of a road traffic accident or heart attack we can be promptly and seamlessly admitted to a first world hospital without having to first locate an insurance document or credit card. These are achievements which we largely take for granted, but which are by no means ubiquitous, even in other wealthy parts of the western world.

However, for all its achievements, the NHS is far from perfect. In my own career, scandal after scandal has rocked this great institution. Alder Hey, the Bristol baby scandal, Shipman, Mid Staffs, Morecambe Bay, Ian Paterson, Gosport and now Telford and Shrewsbury continue to disgrace the wider organisation and make the headlines. There are undoubtedly more to come as well as others that have almost certainly gone under the radar. The common factor in all of these scandals is complacency, a failure to learn, improve and ask critical questions and a determination to cover-up, ignore, deny and carry on in the old way of things, regardless of the cost to our long suffering population. Our most vulnerable patients suffer disproportionately in this respect as was brought home by the Mid Staffs scandal, where funding cuts left many infirm and bedridden patients sitting in their own excrement and drinking from vases. Yet just yards away, NHS managers were congratulating themselves on budgetary savings and their progress towards the great god of 'Foundation Status'.

The NHS's very own figures (almost certainly an underestimate) suggest that some 11,000 patients are lost to avoidable deaths per year, placing us at the very bottom of international league tables for such avoidable disasters. Each one of these is a family left grieving, a wife or husband left alone; children without a parent, parents without a child. Each represents huge and unnecessary suffering and each is by its very definition avoidable.

These figures are nothing short of a national scandal, equivalent to a mid-sized passenger jet crashing for avoidable reasons and killing everyone on board, every week of the year, year after year. Mid Staffs at its very worst cost us up to 1,000 lives over a five year period. The NHS as a whole loses nearly this number to avoidable deaths every month. If a private company were responsible for this loss of life, they'd be closed down instantly, the regulators and the law would be all over them and the press would be baying for prison sentences. Yet we, our politicians and our regulatory bodies are all guilty of utter apathy when it comes to holding our own iconic health service to account for such errors.

THIS STORY IS my own account of life in the NHS. My progress from being an entirely unskilled, immature, stammering, gangly, insecure and acne infested youth, ignorant operating theatre orderly, hapless auxiliary nurse and healthcare assistant, all the way to senior consultant urological surgeon and at one point head of two surgical

NHS departments. It should have been a story ending in destiny fulfilled; an unlikely triumph over the odds; support, respect and companionship from like-minded colleagues. Finally a happy celebration of a career lived according to the best standards of the NHS, culminating in a comfortable retirement, looking back on decades of satisfying service.

That is not the story of this book. My determination to stay true to the founding principles of the NHS led me into direct conflict with the very organisation that I had committed my entire adult life to. Shocked to the core and deeply distressed by some of the lapses of care that I witnessed during my consultant career, I was always clear about my duty to myself, the wider organisation, the regulators and above all else, the patients. I was determined to succeed in driving up standards to levels appropriate to a 21st century NHS. Like so many equally determined individuals before me, I failed and my family have paid very dearly for my efforts.

This book is my story, primarily written for those who wish to gain an insight into the NHS, its attitude to clinical errors and its instinctive reaction towards those who speak up for patients and who discharge their duty of candour. If it achieves anything then I hope that it will act as a catalyst for real change and for a rediscovery of the basic principles of care that once made the NHS the envy of the world. I hope that it will inform its readers about the inability of the current administration to evolve, learn and change for the better. I hope that it will expose the sheer inertia and resistance to improvement that has dogged my consultant career. I hope that it will serve as a wake-up call to NHS regulatory bodies like the Care Quality Commission and NHS Improvement who seem to excel only at being asleep on duty. I hope that it will provoke debate on the adequacy (or not) of current whistle-blower protection, employment law and the kind of impossible position that hard working and well-meaning employees can be placed in, caught between their professional duty on one hand and an oppressive employer with a history of complacency and cover-up on the other.

I hope that my sense of anger and injustice will come across clearly and that my account will help to prevent other families going through the pain of years of separation that my own has had to endure. Above all else, I hope that it will help to inspire those who follow me to firmly move this great but failing organisation back towards its inspirational founding principles and ambitions.

I am determined to place these facts into the public domain in the hope of stimulating a fully informed public debate over NHS clinical safety, corporate governance, efficiency and whistle-blowing. If this account can play a small role in fostering and shaping an NHS which is transparent, open, honest and self-critical; one that can use public funds efficiently and can learn and adapt from its mistakes and one which can listen constructively to those who hold opinions that, for the wider organisation, may be uncomfortable then the ordeal that the NHS continues to put me and my family through will not have been in vain.

PART I

*Career, neglect,
whistle-blowing
and dismissal*

CHAPTER ONE

Vocation

1980: Preston, Lancashire.

LIFE OFTEN SEEMS like little more than stumbling as best we can through a sequence of random, chaotic events, chance encounters and mundane, utterly forgettable days. But sometimes, circumstances that seem at the time like trivial, meaningless coincidences can re-define and totally change our entire lives. Already committed to following my father into a career in retail pharmacy, a throwaway chance exchange between him and a fellow golfer turned my future utterly upside down.

The year was 1980. The fellow golfer was Bob Thomson, previous Captain and future President of Preston Golf Club, larger-than-life character and consultant urological surgeon.

Bob's comment was simple. Why didn't I spend a day in theatre with him at the PRI (Preston Royal Infirmary – long since gone)? My father could have so easily forgotten the exchange, but he didn't and my life was to change forever.

I was eighteen and already into my first year of pharmacy at Bath University. I told my parents with some considerable force and anxiety, 'No! No way, definitely not! I'll hate every minute. I can't stand the sight of blood and I'll throw up or faint or both.'

This was both right and wrong. Whilst I didn't vomit, I certainly fainted spectacularly, going over backwards, cracking my head and having to be carried out of the operating theatre by the anaesthetist and several nurses. Soaked in sweat, I was left to recover on the patient's bed outside whilst Bob finished the circumcision. Bob later remarked that at least I fell the right way; backwards rather than face down into the operation.

Of course, it would never be allowed nowadays, which is a terrible shame. I had absolutely no idea that I had it in me to be a surgeon, and I wonder how many others might have made infinitely better surgeons than me if only they'd also had the chance to experience the rarefied and utterly addictive atmosphere of a modern day operating theatre.

Once I'd got the unmanly act of fainting out of the way, I relaxed, becoming totally transfixed by the experience and overwhelmed with admiration for the tight and disciplined nature of the surgical, anaesthetic and nursing team. Quick and efficient, yet humane and caring, I'd never come across such close-knit group discipline and work ethic. I was in awe of the fact that such intense commitment and concentration was a regular daily thing for these individuals. The atmosphere was tightly focussed yet also relaxed, with everyone seeming to be comfortable with and confident in their role. I felt that I'd come across a truly very special example of compassion and dedication and it made the deepest possible impression on me. The day seemed to fly past in no time, yet simultaneously, time would stand still whilst each operation reached its climax.

Closing my eyes and regressing nearly 40 years, I can still smell the faint odour of anaesthetic agents, sense the concentration, hear the rustle of surgical gowns, the sighing noise of the ventilator and the delicate click of fine surgical steel at work. It seems inconceivable that this was four decades ago.

I still have a treasured memory of Bob that day in his theatre blues during lunch, with his bloodstained white boots propped up on a wooden table in the surgeons' room and his surgical mask dangling round his neck. Dicta-phone in one hand, telephone in the other, secretaries rushing in and out with notes and letters, munching on sandwiches whilst rattling off rapid-fire letters on the dicta-phone, simultaneously fielding endless urgent phone calls, yet carrying off the whole process with effortless precision and humour.

I was entranced, with a sense of absolute destiny and vocation, *I want to be like him!*

Without that chance golf club conversation, everything would have been different. I'd have pursued a career as a retail pharmacist and would never have even known that my future wife and medical school friends-to-be even existed. Our three boys would never have been born and my entire life and extended family would have been totally, utterly different. By the end of the day I was both exhausted and hooked.

I eschewed the buses and walked all the way home from the PRI, deep in thought, without a coat and oblivious to the pouring rain. After arriving home utterly sodden, shivering and footsore, thawing out in the bath and popping several blisters, I told my parents that I now knew what I wanted to do with my life.

I want to be a consultant urological surgeon.

CHAPTER TWO

In limbo

GETTING INTO MEDICAL SCHOOL wasn't easy, but I had at least been given a good start in life. I grew up in North Preston as the oldest of a happy family of four children. My parents, Frank and Jean against some resistance made sure that I did my homework and I'd finished at Cardinal Newman College with four reasonable A levels, going on to study pharmacy at Bath University. Now, suddenly and half way through my first year, everything was utterly changed and, in the short term at least, significantly for the worse.

Having never been very committed to pharmacy, my interest diminished further after my day with Bob. I applied to various medical schools, was (unsurprisingly) turned down and then predictably failed my end-of-year exams. Thankfully, the Dean at Bath University was understanding and tactfully suggested that I took a year out to consider whether I really wanted to do pharmacy. Bob got me a job at a small private hospital called Mount Street Hospital in Preston and I set about trying to get into medical school.

The twelve months from summer 1981-82 was a year of downs and ups. It couldn't have started much more badly. Having failed both to get into medical school and my Bath University exams, I got rather humiliatingly dumped by my then girlfriend. Autumn and winter of 1981 was a very dark and gloomy time indeed and will forever be associated in my mind with failure. Statistically impossible, nevertheless in my memory, the sun never appeared and it never seemed to stop raining for months. Thankfully, my friends and family were hugely supportive and with the dawn of a new year, things looked up. Despite being at the very bottom of the pecking order at Mount Street Hospital, I was gaining experience every day. Working as an unskilled ward orderly, auxiliary nurse and theatre orderly taught me invaluable lessons about patients, the hospital hierarchy and basic nursing and surgical skills. My parents were totally committed to backing my efforts to get into medical school and several consultants at Mount Street were kind enough to write letters and references for me (including Bob and Chris Faulkes, consultant orthopaedic surgeon). In about April/May of 1982 I was offered interviews at Charing Cross and Westminster Medical School, and St Georges Hospital Medical School, both in London.

My final interview question at Charing Cross nearly floored me:

'Well, Mr Duffy. I see that you work at a private hospital. What do you think of private medicine then…?'

I looked in desperation for any clues as to the political allegiances of my questioner. He was male, bland, late-middle aged and wore a tweed jacket and neutral shirt and tie. The jacket could have cost hundreds from Harrods, or been picked up at a charity car boot sale for a fiver. He could have been a Guardian reading medical sociologist and passionate advocate of free healthcare for all or equally a Telegraph reading professor of orthopaedic surgery, earning vast amounts from his London private practice.

Somehow, fear, ambition and adrenaline conspired together and I blurted out,

'I think it's a shame that it's necessary… Sir…'

Thankfully that seemed to do the trick and a few weeks later I opened a letter from Charing Cross and Westminster Medical School, telling me that I had an unconditional place there. A split second later I was engulfed by the family, with hugs, tears, laughter and relief.

It was early summer of 1982 and, somehow, against all the odds, I was in.

CHAPTER THREE

Medical school

I WASN'T VERY POPULAR at medical school, at least not for the first couple of years. Everyone seemed to have superior A levels and accents to mine and I was very intimidated by the high quality southern England private educational backgrounds that some of my contemporaries came from. Worse than that, I had been given an industrial sized lambasting by Lancashire Education Authority for wasting a full years grant after failing at Bath University. It was made crystal clear to me that if I got chucked out of medical school in the same way, there'd be absolutely no further opportunities for higher education.

As a result, whilst everyone else was busy partying and drinking too much alcohol during Freshers' week in the best, finest and most honourable tradition of medical students everywhere; I hid away in the library. Having discovered that we started dissection with the anatomy of the back, I was already engrossed in *latissimus dorsi* and *rhomboideus major*. Needless to say, this didn't do much for my popularity.

Charing Cross and Westminster Medical School had two major student culls, the big one coming at the end of the first year and a lesser chucking out session at the end of the second. Thankfully, and having done little more than study for two years I survived both and enjoyed my anatomy studies enough to embark on an intercalated Batchelor of Science (BSc) degree, adding an extra year to my studies. With the benefit of hindsight, I'm not sure it was really worth it but regardless, I emerged with a 2:1, enjoyed an extra summer holiday, eased off the work, started socialising and enjoying life a little more, moved into new accommodation in Shepherd's Bush and embarked on my three clinical years.

With the glaring exception of psychiatry I liked all my clinical subjects. However it was always surgery that I came back to. I loved all my surgical firms and attachments but without a doubt the most memorable was the privileged, all-too-few weeks that I spent at Westminster Hospital. This was under the tutelage of Professor Harold Ellis CBE, already a famous name amongst medical students and junior doctors as a result of his co-authoring of *Lecture Notes on General Surgery*. He was nevertheless a wonderfully humble, down to earth and inspiring teacher and would think nothing of sitting down with a couple of medical students and teaching us during his free time. I have a vivid memory of being second surgical assistant to him when, with the diseased gall-bladder hanging on by the tiniest thread he handed the scissors to me saying: *There you go, you can call that your first cholecystectomy.*

Even now, more than 30 years on, if I'm a bit stuck with how to manage a difficult situation I still ask myself: *How would Prof' Ellis have handled this?*

The preclinical years bring some gruesome sights, particularly the anatomy dissections but it is during the clinical years where young doctors-to-be really become exposed to the stresses and traumas that go hand in hand with clinical practice. I struggled at times with some of the human suffering, coming home almost sobbing and fighting back tears one evening, after a particularly upsetting paediatric ward round at Ealing Hospital, where I'd encountered several school aged and younger children with terminal cancers. I was deeply moved by their courage and shocked to the core by what seemed to be life's arbitrary and random cruelty. It is difficult to not be traumatised by some of the sights encountered on busy NHS wards, especially when you come upon these things for the first time after a relatively sheltered upbringing.

The failed attempts at a cot death resuscitation of a tiny baby boy in A&E at the West Middlesex Hospital left me utterly distraught and I've never left behind the despairing shriek of the young mother when the news was broken to her. We all heard it through several closed doors and I certainly wasn't the only person to be left traumatised, with several members of staff left in tears afterwards and no one looking anyone else in the eye for hours afterwards.

Similarly, I still have awful memories of a young man bleeding out from oesophageal varices at Redhill Hospital, sometime in the mid 80's. *Varices*, as they're known, are a kind of varicose vein that forms around the lower gullet, often but not always, the result of long term alcohol abuse. If they bleed, the haemorrhage can be terrifying. Thankfully for this patient, he was unconscious by the time the bleeding really got out of control, but I'll never forget the sight of nursing staff frantically running back and forth with bowlfuls of the blood that was pouring out of his mouth whilst the medical and surgical teams desperately squeezed fluids from the transfusion bags into his circulation in a vain and failing attempt to stop his life from ebbing away.

Doctors and nurses are expected to be tough and resilient and to be able to withstand the horrors that sometimes get thrown at us, but it is worth remembering that we're all human. Catch an NHS healthcare worker at a candid and relaxed moment and there's a good chance that they'll also be able to recount horrors and traumas that have stayed with them for the rest of their lives. It's a tough balancing act, remaining caring, sensitive and humane without allowing the daily parade of death and suffering to drag you down into depression and apathy or harden you into disinterest. Not everyone manages it.

Holding things together financially as a medical student was tough too. Medical students in their clinical years don't get university holidays and therefore no time to support themselves financially with holiday jobs. Desperate to keep my overdraft under control and despite an understanding bank manager, I nevertheless found myself at one time holding down a weekend job cleaning the toilets and tables in the staff canteen of Terminal 3 at Heathrow airport whilst simultaneously working nights as either an industrial cleaner or auxiliary nurse at places like Charing Cross itself, Ealing or the West Middlesex Hospitals. It's not easy, holding your daytime concentration together after a series of near-sleepless nights but it was at least good practice for my junior doctor years. I haven't forgotten the kindness of a good number of senior nursing staff, offering to cover for me whilst I sneaked off for a few minutes of precious sleep in the wee-small hours.

It was during those bleary, sleep deprived clinical years in the mid 1980's that I first really got together with Fiona. We'd been friends on and off throughout our time as medical students and, with my intercalated BSc; Fiona had moved a year on. However, we grew very close as I worked through my clinical years, getting engaged during my last year and marrying just after my final exams.

Looking back I realise now how much work and planning Fiona and her parents must have put into the wedding. I was engrossed in my final exams, she was doing her junior house officer jobs and my own parents were 250 miles away. Luckily, despite the fact that my wife-to-be was working ridiculous hours, she and her parents were super organised and the whole wedding day went like clockwork, the two of us jetting off the following day for a fortnight's honeymoon in Singapore and Bali.

CHAPTER FOUR

Marriage and junior doctor jobs

AFTER THE EUPHORIA of getting married, qualifying as a doctor and two weeks of luxury in the Far East, things came down to earth with a vengeance. We returned from our honeymoon in late summer 1988 to married junior doctor accommodation at St Peter's Hospital in Chertsey, Surrey. Fiona was training to be a GP and I was due to start my house-officer year; six months of general medicine and six months of surgery. It was to be a brutal introduction to both medical practice and married life, with conflicting timetables meaning that we sometimes barely saw each other for weeks at a time. Even then we were frequently exhausted. These were the dying days of the notorious 'one-in-two' rota, where juniors worked the regular five days a week, (typically 8am to 6pm) in addition to every other night and every other weekend. It typically meant alternating 80 and 140 hour weeks, one weekend off per fortnight and catching what sleep you could at any possible opportunity. I variously remember snatching a few minutes sleep on A&E trolleys, spare patient beds, wing-back chairs on the stroke ward and even operating tables, only to be jerked awake minutes later by the strident tones of the surgical on-call bleep.

My own alternate weekends on-call during my surgical job began on a Friday morning and ended at perhaps six to seven pm after a full working Tuesday, the entire stretch amounting to around 110 hours continuous on-call work without a break. Even when I had an evening off (every other night), I was frequently too exhausted to drive back home and would sleep in my little cell-like on-call room.

EVERY DOCTOR AND NURSE will see a great deal of death during their careers, something that in ordinary life we are mostly kept protected from. Few front-line staff will reach retirement without witnessing some truly appalling and gruesome deaths but sometimes it is the more dignified deaths that leave the greatest mark. Sitting in close contact with someone during their final moments is a truly humbling, sobering experience and a reminder of what awaits us all.

I do not remember most of the many deaths at which I have been present, but one from my junior house-officer year stands out. It was a very elderly and dignified lady in the Royal Surrey County Hospital, sometime in early 1989. She was around 100 years old. It was evident that she was dying and that carrying out the typical 'cardiac arrest' procedure was pointless and inappropriate. For once, my bleep was quiet and there were no outstanding jobs on the ward. She'd been a witty, appreciative and pin-sharp patient, yet had no relatives and no company and I simply sat quietly with her and held her hand whilst she departed this world with the same dignity in death that she had displayed in life. I really hope that it gave her some comfort and I couldn't help but feel sadness and more than a little anger that such a wealth of accumulated wisdom and knowledge was simply being wiped away.

Here was someone who, as a child and young woman would have seen both some of the greatest human achievements and horrors. The first cars, planes, great ocean-traversing steamships, two world wars and the 'Spanish flu' (not talked about nowadays but nevertheless responsible for the deaths of perhaps up to 100 million human beings). She'd grown up in an era where steam trains, canal barges and the pony-and-trap were the height of travelling sophistication, yet lived through the great age of international travel and globalisation, modern communications, space travel and moon landings, the beginning of the computer age, supersonic flight and so-on. It seemed tragic that so many memories and experiences were about to be lost forever. Yet it was striking that she herself was clearly at peace and showed no fear at her impending death.

Apart from occasions like the above I don't remember much of those early years as a doctor which is a great shame. Above all, there was the constant fatigue and pressure to pass exams. Fiona was progressing well with her plans to be a GP, rotating through A&E, obstetrics and gynaecology, elderly care and psychiatry, picking up her DRCOG and MRCGP exams along the way and becoming a partner in a double-handed GP practice just down the road from our flat in Ottershaw in 1991. The surgery (Ottershaw Surgery) is still there today.

My own surgical career proceeded rather more erratically. Single-mindedly pursuing my surgical ambitions and having to re-apply for a fresh job each time I moved on, I worked my way through a series of six or twelve month jobs in South West London. I worked in A&E at St Peter's Hospital in Chertsey, Surrey, followed by orthopaedic surgery at the Mayday Hospital in Croydon, a year of general surgery at St Helier in Carshalton, also South London and then finished with six months of urological surgery, again at St Helier.

St Helier was known amongst the surgical trainees as 'The Hell-hole', renowned for being busy, underfunded and sometimes overwhelmed. My first real introduction to what awaited me was opening my junior doctors' on-call room door for the first time, only to find the room deep frozen, the window broken and pigeon-shit all over the duvet and pillow.

I slept in my elderly VW Polo that night, waking every 90 minutes to turn the engine on and try to absorb a little heat.

Whilst the window ultimately got repaired and the sheets got washed, things didn't improve much. I remember making the mistake of running a bath after a particularly gruelling shift. Stripping off, I returned only to find a bath full of what looked like Iron Bru, or something worse.

Clinically things were little better. I vividly recall blearily blinking out through sleepless, baggy, bloodshot eyes through the St Helier operating theatre windows across the London skyline as Monday morning's dawn broke. I had just finished a weekend on-call, my fourth appendicectomy of the night and still faced a busy clinic and afternoon day surgery list. Moving on from the sleep deprived twelve months of general surgery to the slightly more sedate pace of the urological surgery department was a real pleasure, helped along by the hands-on teaching and mentoring of my consultant bosses John Boyd and Chris Jones. I felt that I'd come full circle back to where I'd started, with the very thing that had inspired me in the first place – urological surgery.

CHAPTER FIVE

Back to the future
Urological surgery

I'D ENJOYED ALL the other surgical specialities, but there was something rather special about urological surgery. Most of the patients are male (perhaps two thirds) and getting towards or into retirement age. In the early 1990's it seemed that almost every other patient had seen service in the war. I vividly recall brave men who had landed on the Normandy beaches, battled their way through Anzio, ridden dispatch motorcycles up to the front-line in France, frozen on the Arctic Russian convoys, fought behind the Japanese lines with the Chindits or flown Bristol Beaufighters against the German night-time bombing raids. They were all deeply impressive characters, it was a true privilege to be of service to them and, sadly, they are pretty much all gone now.

Another attraction of the speciality is the sheer range and amount of cancer work and the fact that most urological cancers can either be cured or, if not cured then very effectively palliated, often for many years.

Finally, there is the sheer variety of procedures, ranging from huge open operations like radical cystoprostatourethrectomy and ileal conduit formation, a four to five hour bladder cancer operation, even if done by two consultants together to a simple ten minute vasectomy under local anaesthetic. Additionally, urological surgery boasts one of the very first truly minimally invasive operations; TURP (transurethral resection of prostate), performed via an endoscopic instrument passed up the urethra (the water pipe) to enable a male patient to pass urine without struggling or having to resort to the much hated catheter.

I took to urological surgery like a duck to water and thoroughly enjoyed my last six months at *The Hell-hole*, learning pretty much all the basic urological standards that still determine my practice today.

After St Helier, my FRCS exams (Fellowship of the Royal College of Surgeons, a necessary pre-requisite for ongoing surgical training) and a period of locum work, I moved on to Salisbury General Hospital and supervision by Gregor McIntosh, a doubly accredited general and urological surgeon. Working under Gregor's supervision I got to grips with TURPs and expanded my general surgical abilities with some of the bigger general surgical procedures such as laparotomy (an open exploratory operation of the abdomen), Hartmann's procedure (an emergency large bowel operation) and various forms of lower limb amputations.

Every surgeon will have tales of their most challenging operations, but sometimes it is the actual decision to operate that can be most taxing and intimidating. It was at Salisbury whilst I was still covering general surgery that one of my most satisfying but also most frightening operations took place.

It was a 15-18 month old boy, admitted under the paediatric doctors with a raised temperature and sepsis (a potentially life-threatening infection). The paediatricians had worked up the tiny and very ill boy as best they could but could find no source for his infection. He'd continued running high temperatures despite antibiotics and in desperation they asked me to see him, as the general surgical registrar on-call. All I recall was a deeply distressed child, screaming and kicking, with his knees drawn up and clearly critically unwell, with pale and equally distressed parents by his side. I couldn't even get near enough to examine him, far less expect any kind of abdominal scan. However, the paediatricians had pretty much ruled out everything other than an abdominal source for his sepsis.

Appendicitis is rare before two years old, but there are few absolute rules in medicine and surgery and, with a sinking heart, I reluctantly agreed with the paediatric team that he really ought to have an exploratory abdominal operation to see if this was the source of the infection. Gregor was away on holiday and I checked with one of Gregor's colleagues to see if they felt that I was doing the right thing. Being inexperienced in paediatric abdominal surgery I was hoping that they might offer to take the case over, but no such luck.

We got the tiny boy to theatre promptly, but things seemed to be going wrong right from the start. The anaesthetist was clearly very unhappy and struggled for some time to get reliable intravenous access (a drip into the baby boy's veins) and then to get him off to sleep safely. As he was gently placed on the operating table, the anaesthetist made her anxieties clear and once he was reasonably stable, she retired to a corner of the operating theatre to order an emergency 'blue-light' transfer post-operatively to Southampton Hospital's paediatric intensive care unit (ICU). Overhearing her discussing the child's critical condition and his further deterioration under anaesthetic with one of the paediatric ICU consultants, I agonised over my now-irreversible decision to operate. *Have I killed this child? What would happen if my surgical exploration was negative? Would he die on the table?*

Having cleansed the skin and placed the surgical drapes, I steeled myself to take the scalpel proffered by the theatre scrub nurse. *I mustn't let her see that my hands are shaking…*

Any abdominal operation proceeds through several layers of tissue. First the skin, then the subcutaneous fat (situated immediately beneath the skin), then the muscle layers and finally the peritoneum before the abdominal cavity itself is entered.

Even before I'd opened the peritoneum there was tissue oedema (abnormal quantities of fluid, associated with inflammation) and I was able to console myself that, whatever the outcome, at least the decision to operate seemed to have been justified. As I opened the peritoneum and entered the abdominal cavity there was a gush of foul, faecal smelling pus and bits of necrotic (dead) appendix. The tiny child had advanced appendicitis and at least the beginnings of peritonitis (a life-threatening general infection of the abdominal cavity). My own sigh of relief at having found a problem that could be corrected was followed only a minute or two later by the anaesthetist, remarking on how quickly the little boy's condition had improved as soon as the pus had been released. Pus and infection under pressure in any closed body cavity is extremely toxic and releasing it can bring almost immediate clinical improvements. Within another minute or two she was on the phone to Southampton to cancel the ICU bed.

I closed up with a huge sense of relief, bordering on euphoria. In the end, the case had gone really well, but it could all have finished so very differently. It was a salutary reminder of just how suddenly junior and middle grade doctors can be thrust into situations well outside their comfort zone and that carry terrifying responsibilities.

The tiny boy was discharged home sometime around a week later, having made a remarkably quick recovery. I wonder if he is aware of just how close to disaster he came in his first years of life? He's hopefully a fit and healthy mid-20's-year-old by now.

After a year at Salisbury it was time to look to some kind of higher research degree. Salisbury's contacts with Southampton came in useful here and I subsequently found myself working out of the Surgical research unit there, looking into the technique of using intravesical chemotherapy to treat bladder cancer (a technique of putting chemotherapy directly into the bladder in the hope of either treating the cancer or reducing the likelihood of it recurring).

This was a major culture shock. Of all the medical specialities, surgery and anaesthesia run to the most stringent timetables, with ward rounds starting at 7.45am or 8-on-the-dot and weekly timetables planned with military precision. Research work, however, was pretty much entirely un-timetabled and as long as the work got done, no one really bothered too much about what time you turned up or left.

I spent 2½ very different years at Southampton and it probably took a good six months before I really found my feet and adjusted to the demands and expectations of surgical research work. Thankfully my mentor, Dr Alan Cooper was tirelessly patient with me and I hope that I proved to be a good investment in the end. I finally hit my stride in the last 18 months and was rewarded with several publications in scientific journals and podium presentations at the annual BAUS conference (British Association of Urological Surgeons) and the AUA (American Urological Association) in Florida. However, academia never really felt quite right for me and I was very intimidated by the sheer intellect of some of those around me. Presenting and being criticised over your research is *de rigueur* in science and I used to find such lectures utterly terrifying. Paradoxically, the surgical and medical audiences were usually quite tame and forgiving. It was the academic and scientific conferences that were utterly ruthless. I'd dread them for days ahead and you'd never know if someone was going to skewer you with an unanticipated question and mercilessly leave you gasping and wriggling with embarrassment on the podium like a freshly landed fish.

By late 1995 I seemed to have collected enough worthwhile data to write up my MD thesis and started looking around for higher surgical training schemes. Continuing my education in the Salisbury/Wessex/Southampton area appealed as I'd made some good friends and mentors in the area but it would have left me commuting every day from our new house in Surrey. Thankfully, the ideal job came up in South West Thames, based around St George's Hospital Medical School. I applied for higher training in urological surgery and to my delight was accepted, starting work at St George's itself in May of 1996.

My next five years proved to be my making, rotating through St George's, Epsom Hospital, The Institute of Urology (part of University College Hospital, London), St George's again and finally St Peter's in Chertsey, just down the road from where we lived. Each year was special in its own way and I received an outstanding education and preparation for consultant life but perhaps the early year at Epsom was the most memorable. I was desperate to get as much experience as possible under my belt and over the next twelve months and under the watchful supervision of Mike Bailey and Clive Charig I worked my way through hundreds of TURPs and TURBTs (similar to TURPs but performed to remove bladder cancers), ureteroscopies (endoscopic operations on the very tiny and easily damaged tubes draining the kidneys down to the bladder) and other 'core' urological procedures. Keen to get to grips with the bigger stuff, I carried out my first radical nephrectomy (open total surgical removal of a malignant kidney) with Clive Charig, radical prostatectomy for a malignant prostate with Mike Bailey and performed parts of the biggest of the common urological operations, the radical cystectomy (total bladder removal).

Julian Shah, David Ralph and Peter Worth at the Institute of Urology, University College, London and Roger Kirby, Betty Gordon, Ken Anson and Mike Bailey again at St George's followed on and were all outstanding mentors, consolidating my experience at Epsom. I was happy to complete my training and survive my FRCS (Urology) passing out exam with the support of Mr Harvey Hills and the rest of the team at St Peter's in Chertsey. I owe all these outstanding mentors a huge debt of gratitude. I finally finished writing up my MD thesis on bladder cancer in 1999, being rewarded with an MD, Special Commendation and an especially colourful gown and mortarboard hat to wear at the Southampton University passing out ceremony.

Formal medical education is a wonderful thing but there are some lessons that can only be learned the hard way. Just as you begin to get confident, feeling that you're finally in your comfort zone, beyond making snap opinions and embarrassing mistakes and can salvage any slight errors of judgement, medicine has a way of putting you firmly back in your place and teaching you to never ever take anything for granted.

The consultation began straightforwardly enough. A frail elderly man, wheeled into the room by his carer and accompanied by a letter from his GP, announcing that he had a raised PSA (prostate cancer blood test). The patient himself looked exhausted, like little more than thin parchment-like skin stretched over a skeletal frame. He looked as though he'd disintegrate into dust if I so much as sneezed loudly. The carer pushing the wheelchair was however, something else. Her olive skin was flawless and marked her out as one of the recent influx of young overseas nurses, probably from the Philippines I judged, without whom the NHS would collapse instantly. There was plenty of skin on display too. Her nursing uniform looked like it had been designed by Benny Hill in the 1970's and then sprayed on. With a top cut lower than any nurse's uniform that I'd ever seen and the bottom revealing slim, toned legs that wouldn't have disgraced a supermodel, it left little to the imagination. Regretfully I tore my eyes away, focused reluctantly on the patient and shook his proffered hand, being very careful in case it came off in my own.

'Mr Jones. Hello. And this is one of your carers?'

'No', he shook his head, 'that's my wife.'

———————

AS MY CAREER BEGAN to consolidate in the mid 1990's, Fiona and I decided that it was high time to start a family and think about our long term future. Edward was duly born in 1997, followed by Robert in 2000 and we began to think of our future in terms of family and a definitive job for me once I had left behind the insecurity of surgical rotations and constantly having to move jobs every six to twelve months. I'd always felt a vocation to work in either North Lancashire, where I'd grown up and had my first heady experience of surgery with Bob, or in next-door Cumbria, where I'd spent many a happy teenage weekend camping, climbing, canoeing and sailing. A job straddling both would be a dream come true.

It would have been easy to settle in Surrey or South West London and take up a local job, but, even after fifteen years in the south, I still pined for the North West of England and particularly the clean, open spaces, lakes, peaks, sunsets and fresh air of the Lake District, Yorkshire Dales, rolling Bowland Hills and pasturelands of North Lancashire. My future, had I stayed in the South East, would have meant facing some difficult choices. NHS consultant salaries are pretty generous by national standards but we could never aspire to a really nice house in prime suburban, stockbroker belt Surrey, at least not without me immersing myself in private work, which would of course take me away from our new family.

A move 250 miles north offered a chance to fulfil my vocation and an opportunity to trade in our Surrey house for something of rather better value in the north. I was braced for some resistance from Fiona who had grown up only a few miles from where we then lived, but I think that she too could see the advantages of moving to a less expensive part of the country. Having checked out the local schools and costs of private education in Surrey, there was clear attraction in Lancaster, with its state funded and very highly respected boys and girls state grammar schools as well as Ripley St Thomas School, a very highly regarded comprehensive. The local hospital in Lancaster, the Royal Lancaster Infirmary (RLI), part of what is now known as the University Hospitals of Morecambe Bay NHS Foundation Trust (or just UHMB), was a fully-fledged district general hospital, very similar to St Peter's, St Helier, Epsom and Salisbury Hospitals where I had spent my most memorable years of training. Importantly, we'd be situated only fifteen to twenty miles from Preston, where I had grown up and would also be in the midst of my mother's extended farming family, many of whom are still scattered around Lancaster, North Lancashire, West Yorkshire and South Cumbria. Finally, we'd be within twenty minutes' drive of Cumbria and the Lakeland peaks, tarns and valleys in one direction and the Yorkshire Dales in another.

A trip up to my parents and a weekend viewing local estate agents and what seemed to be ludicrously low house prices consolidated our interest and I started putting out feelers, making several trips up to Morecambe Bay and meeting up with Glen Staff and Richard Wilson, the two incumbent urological surgeons in 1999. They seemed pleasant and interested and I confirmed our interest in moving up to the area in the event of a job becoming available. Perfectly reasonably, I was told to get back to them once I'd got my final 'passing-out' surgical exam, the FRCS (Urology) (specialist Fellowship of the Royal College of Surgeons). I cleared this last surgical educational hurdle in late 1999, passing my FRCS (Urology) in Dublin and flying home to Heathrow in style, first class inclusive of champagne and smoked salmon, thanks to a perfectly timed free upgrade.

Without any urological posts coming up in Morecambe Bay in the near future I stayed nearly a year at St Peter's Hospital. There was some interest in me from several London and Surrey hospitals, but my heart was set on working for Morecambe Bay and moving to Lancaster. In autumn of 2000, the Trust decided to offer me a six month NHS locum (temporary) consultant job. This was perfect, giving me time to check out Morecambe Bay's hospitals without being formally committed to them and giving them time to assess my abilities. I left Fiona, Edward and Robert in late 2000, staying with my parents on weekdays at their house in Preston and commuting the 250 miles down to see Fiona and the boys at weekends.

CHAPTER SIX

Consultant at last

STARTING AT MORECAMBE BAY NHS TRUST in October of 2000 was another culture shock. I'd been used to the busy schedules and work ethic of the London teaching hospitals and the South West Thames registrar rotation. Sent to work at Furness General Hospital in South West Cumbria for my first two week locum, I vividly remember turning up at 7.45am and walking into the hospital with the salt-smell blowing in off the Irish Sea and the herring and black-backed gulls wheeling and screaming around me, wondering what the hell I'd got myself into.

It all seemed a world apart from London and Surrey, rumbling tube trains and 747's with the occasional Concorde whistling overhead. I was on the ward on the dot of 8am but I needn't have bothered. 'Oh, he'll still be fast asleep in bed,' I was told by a rather surprised staff nurse after asking the whereabouts of the urology junior doctor, 'we'll probably see him sometime after nine...'

Furness General proved a warm, welcoming and a thoroughly pleasant place to work but it didn't take much time for me to develop some reservations about a new colleague. Mr Madhra had been appointed in early 2000 and hence I hadn't met him on my previous visits in 1999. He was on annual leave for two weeks and therefore the first fortnight of my locum was covering for him.

I was asked to go and see the wife of a patient of his on the ICU (Intensive Care Unit) during my first morning. The patient himself was on a ventilator (an artificial breathing machine) when I went up to the unit but I was able to speak to his wife. I clearly remember her terrible distress over her husband's predicament as we sat, discussing his case in the relatives' room. He had undergone a private radical prostatectomy (an operation to remove a malignant prostate) carried out by Mr Madhra but had bled afterwards, requiring a large blood transfusion and having to be returned to theatre at least twice to try and arrest the haemorrhage. In the end one of the vascular consultants had to tie off his internal iliac arteries (the main arteries that supply the pelvic organs with blood) in order to stop the bleeding. I was concerned about such a poor outcome from the operation but what I found really shocking was the pre-operative build up. The family hadn't, in my opinion, been given sufficient accurate or detailed information to help them decide between the different treatments for prostate cancer and had been given the impression that the cancer could be quickly fatal. They'd also been told that the wait for cancer surgery at FGH was a minimum of six months and the patient's wife volunteered that this was why they had paid to go privately, in order to avoid the six month wait on the NHS. This concerned me even more as the private operation had seemingly taken place during Mr Madhra's regular NHS operating list.

Having checked with the secretaries that I'd got my facts right I took myself off to Richard Wilson, the then clinical lead for urology to present my concerns, both about the six month wait for cancer surgery and the performing of major private cancer procedures on NHS operating lists. He fully agreed with my concerns, commenting dryly 'That didn't take you long…'

It wasn't much later that I attended my leaving party down in Surrey. A good number of my old colleagues and trainers came along and I remember a very flattering speech from Mike Bailey, the person that I'd spent the most time with as a trainee and my mentor from both Epsom and St George's. It gave me a good opportunity to have a confidential chat with my ex-trainers about some of the concerns that I'd been having about Mr Madhra. They were all very sympathetic of my predicament and asked if I really felt that I'd made the correct choice of NHS employer. I was warned (even at this early stage) about the career dangers of retaliation and counter-allegations if I reported my concerns to the Trust. Too often, I was told, it falls to a conscientious employee to flag up safety or probity related issues. Subsequently perceived as being a threat or non-team player by both NHS management and colleagues, it is all too common for such a diligent worker to find themselves subject to the wrath of both groups, with management and colleagues all having a vested interest in keeping things quiet and under cover. I was also cautioned about the potential for a racism allegation, being warned that the NHS's knee-jerk response to such allegations tends to be *guilty until proven guilty*.

On the other hand, I was also unequivocally told that I had an absolute duty to bring these issues to the NHS's attention and was also advised that to fail to do so would be a breach of my professional duties and could jeopardise my own career.

They were, of course, all to be proved right in every one of these concerns.

I settled in quickly to my new job and relished the challenge of trying to get waiting times down. Glen Staff and Abul Kamal were running the service out of the Royal Lancaster Infirmary and I largely concentrated on Furness General Hospital during my first year or so. One of the biggest problems was our wait for outpatient appointments. In 2018-19 we complain about waits but it is easy to forget that in 2000 there was an eighteen month wait in some specialities for a regular outpatient appointment. Thankfully, after a year or so we'd got this down to little more than a few weeks.

In 2001, William, our third son was born. We purchased a dream house just down the road from the Royal Lancaster Infirmary and I settled into what seemed to be the perfect life with Fiona and our young family. Despite early struggles with wet and dry rot in our Victorian house, we soon came to love it and it proved the perfect place for our family to grow up. It was situated within walking distance of the local schools, Lancaster city centre and the hospital, boasting a gorgeous hillside garden with a big lawn for the boys and our new kitten to play on and views out over Morecambe Bay, Lancaster Castle and the distant Cumbrian mountains. My parents and old school friends were one stop down the motorway, we were surrounded by farming relatives, I was doing the job that I loved and felt a true vocation for and it seemed that life just couldn't get any better.

Despite my euphoria at the way that things had worked out I distinctly remember moments of trepidation about my future. Whilst there wasn't a cloud on the horizon at that point of my career, I couldn't help wondering about the longer term. In perhaps 2003 whilst the children were still tiny I clearly recall standing out on our lovely balcony, watching the sun set over Heysham and Morecambe Bay, with the Barrow shipyards far on the horizon and the Lakeland hills slowly sinking into the evening mist. I felt a sudden trepidation and fear for all of this that I loved and for my still young family. *How would this end?* I had a sudden premonition and I still recall that chilling moment clearly.

Nothing lasts forever, and I speculated silently about how this happiness and fulfilment would finish. Not well, I sensed. Perhaps with the boys (now peacefully sleeping) growing up and moving away, my parents passing away and perhaps ultimately with Fiona and I growing too old and frail to maintain such a grand and lovely house. Never could I possibly have conceived that things would end far sooner and more punitively, with a sustained and vicious witch-hunt, career ending allegations and my brutal expulsion from the home, family and NHS Trust that I loved and had such a vocation to serve. Neither could I have guessed the role that some of my future colleagues would play in my career demise, colleagues who, at least in part, owed their very appointments and jobs to me.

I shivered and went inside to check on the boys, and the moment passed.

––––––––––––

GLEN STAFF RETIRED in about 2002 and I moved over to the RLI to take over Glen's patients and practice. He'd run a tight ship and it was a challenge living up to his hard work. Luckily, I was able to avail myself of the services of Mr Abul Kamal, Glen's excellent associate specialist. Kamal, as he was known, was indispensable to me, not only for his wide ranging knowledge of both urological surgery and general surgery but also for his knowledge and wisdom about the RLI in which he had worked for many years.

After Glen's retirement and with Kamal's help I set about trying to make inroads into the waiting times in much the same way as I'd done in Furness General Hospital (FGH) in Barrow. It was a busy time, as I also took over Glen's sessions at the Westmorland General Hospital (WGH), at Kendal, whilst retaining some operating time at FGH.

It didn't happen often, but I recall completing a radical cystoprostatourethrectomy and ileal conduit operation one Monday morning at Lancaster with Kamal. This involves the removal of the bladder, prostate and urethra (water-pipe) and diverting the urine to drain via the intestine (bowel) through an outlet known as a stoma into a plastic bag attached to the skin. Finishing up after having removed the patient's cancerous bladder and walking with the patient and anaesthetist round to the Intensive Care Unit, I left the patient's immediate post-op care in Kamal's very capable hands, leapt into the car, raced to Barrow and carried out a similar radical cystoprostatectomy with Richard Wilson in the afternoon at FGH, getting back at maybe 9-10pm. It was a high pressure, full on time but, looking back it was also a generally happy and productive period and I settled into my new role, predominantly based at Lancaster but with regular sessions at FGH and WGH.

Being praised at a North West England audit for the quality and results of our radical cystectomies in Morecambe Bay, by the mid-2000's it seemed that, at last, I'd achieved my lifetime's ambition to be a competent and useful consultant urological surgeon in a part of the country that I'd always wanted to raise a family in.

In the meantime, however, my concerns over clinical standards persisted and I had a number of conversations with senior medical staff between the years of 2001 and 2006. These concerns all related to Mr Madhra and there were several recurring themes. On-call availability was an issue. Another was the sheer number of patients being listed for procedures that I considered unnecessary. Finally, there seemed in my opinion to be a relentless promotion of private work.

Dick Wilson, Abul Kamal and I were all fastidious about arranging our annual leave and would take extreme care to ensure that we swapped cover for our annual leave to make sure that the Trust always had a urological surgeon on-call for emergencies. However, I grew thoroughly sick and tired of receiving calls when I wasn't on duty, telling me that there was an emergency, Mr Madhra was on-call, but was either uncontactable or overseas on a conference or holiday and *I-know-you're-not-on-call-but...* It reached a point where, whenever Mr Madhra was on-call, I'd make sure that I was at home, available and with my mobile phone turned on as it was almost certain that I'd get called over some issue.

Things really came to a head from 2002 on. Firstly, we had yet another case of on-call unavailability involving a seriously unwell diabetic patient in his 40's. This was followed soon after by a second issue over a series of prostate biopsies and Mr Madhra's ability to carry these out to the requisite standards.

Reading back through some of the correspondence some sixteen years later, I was clearly struggling to square my loyalty to the patients and general quality of service with the NHS expectation that I would always support a colleague and his family. One of my earlier letters clearly illustrated my dilemma, with the document clearly stating my anxieties over the consequences for Mr Madhra and his family as well as detailing the fact that I'd agonised over sending it for some three months.

The issue of the diabetic patient was arguably the worst of the individual clinical errors of neglect during this period. It arose on a Sunday, the first inkling of trouble being an urgent lunchtime phone conversation with the senior sister on ward 30 (in those days the combined general surgery and urology ward). The diabetic patient in question had been admitted a day or two earlier with scrotal swelling, pain and redness. This was being treated with antibiotics but on the evening before, things had taken a major turn for the worse and the patient had developed a black patch of necrotic (dead) gangrenous skin on his scrotum.

This is a potentially catastrophic development and is indicative of a condition-called Fournier's gangrene or necrotising fasciitis, more commonly known in the media as a 'flesh eating bacterial infection'. In essence, it is usually several different bacteria all working in conjunction, creating a fast spreading and rapidly lethal form of gangrene. It can happen anywhere in the body, but the scrotum seems particularly vulnerable, particularly in frail and unwell patients. Diabetics seem especially predisposed to this condition.

Mr Madhra had been contacted by the surgical senior house officer (SHO) and registrar the previous Saturday late afternoon/early evening. Both of the surgical doctors had promptly and correctly diagnosed and clearly documented the condition including the conversation with Mr Madhra which included the terms Fournier's gangrene/necrotising fasciitis. It was documented that Mr Madhra had correctly instructed that the patient be started on metronidazole (an antibiotic used in Fournier's gangrene), stating that he would drive over to the hospital to see the patient.

Fournier's gangrene is a mercifully rare problem in urology. I've perhaps operated on eighteen to twenty cases in 25 years. It spreads rapidly, killing the tissues as it goes, often causing considerable pain as well as redness, heat and swelling. In the more fulminating and aggressive cases you can almost see the margins of the infection spreading out through the surrounding skin.

It seems to be a condition of spreading sepsis that causes the blood vessels to clot or 'thrombose', meaning that, whilst antibiotics may slow it down, the drugs can't effectively get to the infected tissues and hence the infection can continue to spread, cutting off the blood supply along its advancing edges as it goes. The only solution to avoid an untimely and horrible death is immediate, emergency surgery to remove all the infected tissue, and even then, mortality rates in some studies approach 50% or more.

I was blissfully unaware of this developing disaster, having passed a quiet Saturday evening with my family and Sunday morning mowing the lawns and looking forward to one of Fiona's excellent Sunday roasts. The news came through from the ward sister just as Fiona was serving up. Mr Madhra hadn't turned up the previous night, she'd been trying to contact him all morning and he wasn't answering his mobile. She told me that when she had gone off duty the previous day the patient had had a small coin sized gangrenous patch. By this point (nearly twenty hours later) he had extensive lower abdominal, scrotal and groin tissue gangrene which was also now extending back around his perineum (skin behind the scrotum) and anus.

I vividly recall Fiona standing with a plate of lunch in each hand, frozen and wide-eyed. She'd heard the conversation and, as an experienced GP she knew exactly what was unfolding.

I asked the surgical sister to contact theatres and the Intensive Care Unit for immediate surgery, apologised profusely to my family and leapt into the car. Luckily, even though I was only two-minute drive from the RLI, an excellent anaesthetic registrar was already standing over the patient by the time that I got there and we agreed to wheel him straight up to theatre ourselves, not waiting for the porters, put the patient to sleep and proceed with emergency debridement (surgical removal of all the infected and gangrenous tissue) there and then. It is a measure of our anxiety that we agreed not to wait for emergency blood tests results to come back and instead felt that emergency surgery should go straight ahead. Performing anaesthesia and major surgery without up to date blood tests is a calculated gamble. Deranged blood electrolytes (sodium, potassium etc.) or anaemia (a low blood haemoglobin condition) can make anaesthesia very hazardous and, from a surgical point of view it is also essential to check that that the patient's blood clotting isn't too deranged in case the patient haemorrhages uncontrollably. Clotting defects and electrolyte disturbances can happen with necrotising fasciitis but neither the anaesthetist nor I felt that we could wait the 30 to 60 minutes for emergency 'bloods' to come back. Instead we agreed to gamble bearing in mind the severity of the situation, starting emergency surgery and correcting any biochemical, haematological or clotting issues *on the table*.

I began to carry out the most extensive debridement that I have ever had to perform on any patient, excising (removing) the whole scrotum, all the perineum to behind the anus, upper thighs, a lot of the skin on the penile shaft and a significant amount of lower abdominal skin before I had cleared all the dead and gangrenous tissue. Mercifully, all seemed quiet and under control at the top end of the operating table (flurries of activity and raised voices at the anaesthetic end of an emergency operation seldom bode well for the patient). Towards the end of the operation I began to feel hopeful that we'd at least given the patient a fighting chance, despite the shock of the surgical team at the sheer extent of the tissue that I'd had to cut away, revealed as I stepped back from the patient.

There is a particular smell to necrotising fasciitis. Medicine and surgery involve exposure to all kinds of noxious smells and offensive odours but there is something horribly toxic, even evil, about the smell given off by the rotting and necrotic flesh in a case of Fournier's gangrene. It is almost impossible not to gag when the smell is strong and, once smelled, it is never forgotten. In other cases, I've actually been able to detect the smell as I've walked into the hospital and make the diagnosis before I've even arrived on the ward. To me, it smells of death itself and the smell gets into everything.

Thankfully, by the end of the operation, both the wound and the air seemed clean and the smell had almost gone, the bowls full of putrid material having been whisked away by the theatre nurses.

Hopefully, we hadn't left any of the infected tissues behind.

The extent of the surgery was too great to wake the patient up and he was transferred to ICU post-operatively for continued anaesthesia, ventilation and monitoring.

Mr Madhra finally turned up on ward 30, mid-afternoon in his golfing clothes.

It took many weeks until we were finally able to get the patient out of the RLI. For the first few days we transferred him on a daily basis from the Intensive Care Unit, still on a ventilator for his repeat wound inspections, further debridements of any suspicious looking tissues and dressing changes. He was finally woken up and transferred to the ward several days later.

Of course, the nursing staff then had to try to manage him with wounds that were open and raw. Fournier's gangrene rarely affects the testicles themselves as they have a different blood supply from the skin in the area and hence it wasn't necessary to remove them. However, both were left fully exposed and without skin cover.

These kinds of wounds leak fluid copiously and dressings rapidly get sodden and infected. Hence the patient had to have regular daily dressing changes which were screaming agony for him. The extent of the debridement was horrifying to us all, looking as though the patient had had several shark bites taken out of him and it was clearly never going to be possible to close the wounds. Ultimately, he would require extensive skin grafting, the preserve of the plastic surgeons. However, it is a necessary pre-requisite that the wound is mature, clean and healthy prior to grafting, with a layer of *granulation tissue* (a kind of inflammatory response from the body) so that the grafted skin can 'take'.

It took many weeks to reach this position. I tried placing the testicles into thigh pouches to protect them, (beneath the skin of the groin) but too much thigh skin had been excised so we had no choice but to leave them raw and without any skin cover. Up until then, as the sole urology consultant at RLI, I went in to see the patient every day, seven days a week on ward 30 whether I was on-call or not and changed his dressings using a mixture of morphine, midazolam (a sedative) and Entonox (laughing gas) as a kind of amateur anaesthetic to try and relieve the poor patient's agony. Sister Michelle Holmes deserves a special mention here. She bore the brunt of the patient's intensive nursing needs during this period and we got into a routine where I'd phone ahead, Michelle would give the intravenous morphine about ten minutes ahead and I'd drip-feed in the midazolam and more morphine whilst the patient used the Entonox mask.

To this day I am amazed that this man survived. He was unbelievably stoical where many patients (probably myself included) would have turned their face into the pillow and given up. He fought like a tiger to survive and never once complained, despite his excruciating agony. Michelle and I were ultimately rewarded for our efforts when, weeks later, he was finally judged to be stable enough and fit to be accepted by the Preston plastic surgeons, being transferred to the Royal Preston Hospital for extensive skin grafts.

I was lucky enough to meet the patient again, several years later, in a chance encounter outside the outpatient department which he was attending as a part of his diabetic follow-up. We shook hands and embraced with real warmth. Luckily he seemed to remember little of his suffering during those awful weeks. The human mind seems to have a remarkable ability to block out such terribly traumatic events and I was truly delighted to see him looking so well. My own psychology has been less successful in suppressing those memories and he is one of several cases that I still have nightmares about, waking up in a sweat, hearing him screaming into his Entonox mask and smelling that horrific anaerobic gangrenous smell, something that persisted on my hands for days after, despite wearing two layers of surgical gloves.

———————

HAVING ALREADY COMMUNICATED a number of other significant concerns to management I felt that I had no choice but formally flag this clinical failing up to the senior medical hierarchy.

A face-to-face meeting was the consequence and, sadly, a typical NHS response was the outcome. Mr Madhra insisted that the diagnosis handed over to him was 'epididymitis', a relatively unaggressive alternative diagnosis, treated with antibiotics only and not requiring of emergency surgery. It was clearly documented in the notes that the diagnosis handed over was Fournier's gangrene/necrotising fasciitis (neither of which sounds remotely like epididymitis over the phone) and there was a documented instruction from Mr Madhra to start the patient on metronidazole (a key antibiotic for the treatment of necrotising fasciitis and never used in epididymitis) but nevertheless Mr Madhra received nothing more than a mild admonishment from the senior medic in question and an instruction to 'Get yourself out and deal with it next time....'

There were numerous other ongoing issues at the time including what I considered to be significant numbers of patients being listed for inappropriate or unnecessary operations and excessively large waiting lists. There were also ongoing issues over on-call availability and the promotion of private work, but the next really big one was Mr Madhra's prostate biopsy technique. I'd been thoroughly taught this technique myself by Clive Charig at Epsom back in 1996. The aim was to sample the prostate with a minimum of eight (nowadays at least twelve) biopsies, each one aimed at a separate area of the prostate and using an ultrasound scanner to guide the needle. Done adequately, it is all but impossible to miss the prostate, even with one biopsy.

We acquired a prostate biopsy ultrasound machine in about 2003. Both Kavinder Madhra and I began using it on a regular basis. Almost immediately I began to get calls from the secretaries and urology nursing staff reporting that some or all of Mr Madhra's prostate biopsies had little or no prostate in them. Initially disbelieving of this, I subsequently spoke to the laboratory technicians. Having established the fact that several of Mr Madhra's prostate biopsy specimens did indeed contain nothing more than bits of bowel, fat and connective tissue, I once again passed my concerns up to the senior medical hierarchy. Once again we had a face to face meeting where I was bluntly told that this was just bad luck, happens to everyone and that my concerns were purely motivated by prejudice.

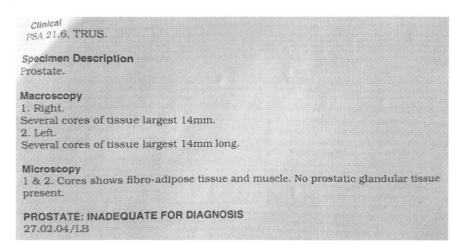

Clinical
PSA 21.6, TRUS.

Specimen Description
Prostate.

Macroscopy
1. Right.
Several cores of tissue largest 14mm.
2. Left.
Several cores of tissue largest 14mm long.

Microscopy
1 & 2. Cores shows fibro-adipose tissue and muscle. No prostatic glandular tissue present.

PROSTATE: INADEQUATE FOR DIAGNOSIS
27.02.04/LB

In 2004 we appointed Carl Rowbotham. Carl and I had gone through the South West Thames training rotation together and I was very flattered to be approached by such a good candidate regarding the possibility of a job. Carl was duly appointed and took over some of my Lancaster sessions as well as the bulk of the Kendal work. He too quickly declared his unease over some of the clinical standards in the department.

Richard Wilson was the senior urological surgeon at the time and after he also expressed concerns, we had another meeting at the Westmorland General Hospital with Kavinder Madhra, Richard Wilson, myself and the Medical Director. Initially making no progress and with Mr Madhra vehemently and indignantly protesting his competence and superior knowledge of the procedure to mine, halfway through the meeting I had a sudden thought. We had a prostate biopsy ultrasound scanner just down the corridor. *Could Mr Madhra demonstrate his technique to us?*

After furious protests my suggestion prevailed and I wheeled the machine into the meeting room, plugged it in and invited Mr Madhra to demonstrate his technique. It was excruciating to watch. I had to show him where the 'on' switch was located, how to load up the software, how to connect the probe, how to measure the prostate size and, most crucially, how to bring up the digital guide which showed the operator where the needle went in the prostate. By the end, the Medical Director was sitting with his head in his hands and there was no doubt over what needed to be done.

Over the next six weeks, Carl Rowbotham and I spent every free half day, unpaid, recalling every negative biopsy patient of Mr Madhra's, explaining to them what had happened and repeating their biopsies, several of the patients subsequently proving to have prostate cancer.

Still ongoing at this point was an investigation into another disaster, with a middle aged lady presenting to Mr Madhra with recurrent cystitis (bladder infection), yet inexplicably being listed for a complex and unnecessary operation for incontinence. Having undergone a 'rectus sheath sling' procedure and being unable to pass urine postoperatively, the poor patient had to be taught to pass a catheter (a bladder drainage tube) several times a day in order to empty her bladder.

At this point I was informed by the then Medical Director that Mr Madhra's complaints folder was bigger than all the other consultants in the Trust put together and was bluntly told by the then chief executive that he'd have sacked me 18 months earlier if I'd behaved similarly.

With many other incidents and errors being reported it was now inevitable that matters would have to be reviewed externally.

After the intervention of the National Clinical Assessment Service (NCAS), similar to the General Medical Council (GMC), Mr Madhra was suspended and after at least a year of senior management dithering, he was sent off for retraining.

At the time, I felt a mixture of guilt that my intervention had caused such problems for a colleague and his family, but also relief that my concerns had been finally been addressed. I looked forward with real optimism to much improved clinical standards in the urological surgery unit at Morecambe Bay. In the longer term I couldn't have been much more wrong.

CHAPTER SEVEN

Peak practice

OTHER THAN THESE ISSUES my job proceeded well. Having been promoted to clinical lead of the urological surgery department in 2003, I was greatly helped in my desire to keep driving up standards by the support of Richard Wilson, followed by Carl Rowbotham's appointment and also the subsequent appointment of both Colin Cutting and Debbie Skennerton in 2006-7. Debbie and Colin had also trained with me in South West Thames and were extremely valuable additions to the department, although Debbie never really settled into the job, preferring to move back to the south east of England a year or two later to take up a post at Epsom, where I'd done my first full registrar year. She was (and still is) much missed for her commitment and for bringing a refreshing common sense female presence to a department otherwise largely dominated by males.

One of the big changes brought in after Carl Rowbotham's appointment was the concept of the 'one-stop clinic'. These are relatively common now (but perhaps not as common as they ought to be) and were a great success for us. The original concept came out of a conversation between Carl and myself shortly after his appointment. We were talking about the excellent quality of the GP referrals locally and the fact that it was usually possible to know in advance which tests the patients would need even before they walked into the clinic room. We were not impressed with the new *two week wait* (2ww) political cancer target, requiring us to see all possible cancers within two weeks of referral. We agreed that most 2ww referrals weren't cancer, and most cancers that we found didn't come through the new 2ww pathway. There must be a better way. After some bouncing around of ideas and putting all of these thoughts together, the concept of a one stop clinic emerged where we'd see _everyone_ within two weeks (hence meeting the two week target) and get all the primary diagnostic tests (ultrasound, endoscopy, prostate biopsies etc.) at the first visit. These would be organised in advance on the basis of the referring letter, followed by a consultation at the same visit with the results of these tests, as far as was possible.

Carl really got the bit between his teeth over this and disappeared off to check how other cutting edge departments were doing things. Returning with a well thought out business plan, it was instantly and frustratingly dismissed by senior managers as being 'unworkable'.

In 2006 there was a big proposed change in the regional care structures. In both Lancashire and Cumbria the private sector was pushing hard to take work away from the NHS and at one point we were told that the private sector wanted to take 80% of the straight-forward and profitable diagnostics, elective (non-emergency) operating and referrals. Privately run community assessment and treatment service (CATS) centres were proposed and Morecambe Bay's senior managers went into a blind panic, faced with the possibility of being stripped of all our profitable services and left only with the loss making emergencies and the sick, elderly patients that the private centres didn't want. The only option was to show that we could do it better than CATS. Carl's plan was taken off the shelf, dusted down and we were told 'Just do it! Cost is no object. The sooner the better. How about yesterday for a start date?'

In the end we set what seemed to me to be hopelessly optimistic start dates but senior management were unstoppable. No prisoners were taken and by the end of 2006 we had a one-stop clinic running out of Kendal, rapidly followed by Lancaster and Barrow. They are still running today and enabled me (as clinical lead) to spend my evenings doing the rounds of the local and regional public and private meetings relating to CATS, speaking out about the fact that we could do things much better than the private sector was propos-ing and generally performing a rear-guard action against the advancing threat. In the end, the private sector threat to the Trust was seen off and it is a salutary lesson in what the NHS can do if suitably incentivised.

We linked these rapid diagnostic clinics up with other innovations like 'pooled waiting lists' and 'rapid turnover operating lists'. By carefully selecting both staff and patients and planning ahead to ensure maximum usage of facilities, we were able to operate on up to twelve patients per list rather than the usual four. There was a wonderful 'all hands on deck' feeling in those days (less than 10 years ago, although it seems a lifetime away to me now), with everyone pulling in the same direction and a sense of real progress and momentum behind the department.

Staying behind on the odd evening after work to do extra unpaid clinics and operating lists, as well as heading in on Saturday mornings to do the same just seemed natural and appropriate. Waiting times tumbled, the department was bringing in large financial surpluses for the Trust, senior management all the way up to Tony Halsall, the then chief executive, seemed to be fully behind us and, despite the sad resignation of Debbie Skennerton part way through this; it really felt that we were on a roll.

In 2008 the department won a prestigious award from Hospital Doctor magazine for the 'National Clinical Lead of the Year' as a consequence of the above innovations and we were asked by the Cumbria Primary Care Trust (PCT) to roll out our model of urology across North Cumbria, a neighbouring Trust whose urology department was struggling with the workload.

For about six months I became clinical lead of their department too as well as carrying on with the clinical lead work for my home Trust in Morecambe Bay. The front-line staff of Carlisle, Penrith and Whitehaven were every bit as committed as those from Morecambe Bay and we received much positive feedback from patients, staff and GPs in North Cumbria for opening up more one-stop clinics in Penrith and Workington. Towards the end of this period we were poised to open up further clinics in Carlisle, Whitehaven and Keswick when the funding for the initiative suddenly collapsed in the spending squeeze that came in roughly 2009. The locum who was being employed to back-fill some of my sessions in Lancaster was dismissed and, after struggling on through summer, trying to do two full time clinical jobs at once and without any ring-fenced time to do my double clinical lead work too, I very regretfully had to pull out of these projects in North Cumbria. Sadly and within days, all of our achievements were swiftly closed down.

In the meantime we did however still manage to open up a variant of these clinics called 'community one stop clinics' in both Garstang and Morecambe. The urology team would travel out to Primary Care Centres, taking the latest hospital diagnostic technology (portable ultrasound scanners and endoscopy equipment) with them in the back of an estate car. To the best of my knowledge, the clinic in Morecambe is still going.

Looking back to 2008-9, there is really no doubt that this is where my career peaked. From this point on with a brief but welcome respite when I transferred back to Furness General Hospital in Barrow, things seemed to accelerate unstoppably downwards. I'm still not sure, even with the benefit of hindsight, how I could have avoided this without betraying my professional instincts and obligations.

CHAPTER EIGHT

Old, ugly and experienced –
Things start to deteriorate

BY 2010 I'D BEGUN to have some qualms about the Trust. Having always nurtured the ambition to be appointed to South Lakes/North Lancashire, my loyalty to the Trust knew no bounds for my first decade of service. However, as the noughties drew to a close, my confidence in the Trust's overall standards began to wobble. It was clear that Morecambe Bay Hospitals was coming under huge pressure to achieve the new status of being a 'Foundation Trust' and it was made equally clear by the Department of Health that any laggards would ultimately be taken over by other Trusts. Morecambe Bay was in a particularly vulnerable position, using three hospitals to serve a small population of only around 250,000 as a consequence of the dispersed rural population in North Lancashire and South Cumbria. There was no chance of closing two of the three hospitals and it was self-evident that the Trust would have to try and struggle on with three hospitals to run but only one hospital's worth of funding. The logical managerial response to the need to balance budgets was to try and slash costs and spending and the consequences soon showed through in the staffing levels on the wards. After speaking out on several occasions, I began submitting emails, detailing my concerns. Well aware of the breaking news about the clinical and management errors characterising the Mid-Staffordshire NHS Trust, I was deeply troubled that we appeared to be making the same mistakes in Morecambe Bay.

'Mid Staffs' as it became known was a major scandal at about this time and those of us who worked in the health service were well aware of the immense pressure on all NHS Hospitals during this period. To secure their futures, hospitals were expected to maintain financial balance amongst other things, thereby achieving 'Foundation Status'. Those who were unable to manage this seemed doomed to being taken over by neighbouring, more successful Trusts. Any member of the executive of one of these struggling hospital groups would have faced the real prospect of an abrupt end to their career aspirations in the event of such an outcome. As a result, there was a ruthless drive to cut expenditure, hastily paper over any clinical cracks that might be appearing and portray an image of smoothly run, slick and efficient hospital at all costs. This is, of course, the trap that Mid Staffs fell into and somewhere between 400 and 1,000 patients over a fifty month period paid the ultimate price for it.

Acutely aware of these developing issues and after much agonising I stood down as clinical lead in mid-2010. I felt that, having spoken out without success about my concerns, I should formally register such concerns by removing myself from the management team. I was not the only one to express my concerns about clinical standards within the Morecambe Bay. A small group of courageous consultants also pressed the Trust with their concerns at around this time, submitting a detailed document to the Board about clinical and corporate governance. Tellingly, very few if any of this group of consultants still survive in the Trust and when I ultimately lost my job, I was one of the last remaining ones who had clearly spoken out during this era.

I continued to work as a full time consultant urological surgeon and was replaced as clinical lead by Mr Colin Cutting. My concerns and those of others who also found themselves having to move on from Morecambe Bay were, of course, fully vindicated by the publication of the Morecambe Bay Report into the Trust by Dr Kirkup in March 2015, although I doubt if this will offer those brave colleagues much comfort.

The urology department underwent some major changes in the late 2000's. Richard Wilson took a rather sudden and unexpected retirement despite our efforts to try and persuade him to stay on. Debbie Skennerton had resigned a year or two earlier and moved to a new job in Epsom and Kamal was making it clear that he was now seriously considering a well-earned retirement, although we managed to persuade him to continue part time for another year or two.

In response, we recruited two more consultants, Mr Jain and Mr Naseem, and at about this point Mr Madhra was fully reinstated.

I had no concerns about Mr Jain's appointment, or Mr Naseem's. In fact, I'd sat on Mr Naseem's interview committee which, at the end of the interview was divided over whether to appoint or not. After prolonged discussions and vigorous debate, Colin Cutting and I were both strongly in favour of appointing Mr Naseem and our views prevailed. At the time I anticipated no future problems.

Similarly, Mr Jain had been appointed to his locum job by me in the dying days of my clinical leadership. At an informal interview he had acknowledged a historical problem with the GMC, but told me that it was 'a misunderstanding' and had been cleared up with 'no case to answer'. Foolishly, I took this assurance at face value and after appointing him as locum consultant he went on to be offered a formal post by Colin Cutting after I'd stepped down from the clinical lead job. Only years later and after a tip off from a patient complainant did I realise that, according to the patient and a newspaper article, Mr Jain had in fact been investigated by the GMC for serious professional misconduct and falsifying aspects of his CV, including his age, experience, qualifications and publications. Had I been aware of this, I'd never have even invited him for interview.

I was, however, more nervous about Mr Madhra's reinstatement after his retraining. No evidence was offered to the department to convince us that there'd been any change in attitude or insight, and I was even more concerned to receive a phone call from a member of the public late one evening, warning me that Mr Madhra was openly talking about how he intended to inflict his revenge on me for expressing my concerns about his clinical standards.

Recalling the conversation with my ex-trainers in London all those years earlier together with the previous *guilty-until-proven-guilty* warnings from before Mr Madhra's suspension, I took my concerns about retaliation to the then Medical Director of the Trust.

As a consequence, two employment law solicitors were asked to come to the RLI and brief me on my concerns. I clearly remember being bluntly told by the dominant, rather portly and clearly more senior and important partner, 'Look, if you choose to report clinical negligence then you must expect the inevitable retaliation. As a consultant surgeon yourself, you're old, ugly and experienced enough to be able to take it and if you can't, then keep quiet!'

I quietly vowed that, no matter how old or ugly, I would never be silenced over serious clinical errors and neglect. *Ever!*

Looking back, my stepping down as clinical lead was probably the tipping point. In career terms I think that I was perhaps regarded as someone with potential but also someone who was lacking in killer instinct, ruthless ambition and self-promotion. In speaking out against the then obsession with achieving Foundation Status I had marked myself out as someone who didn't always slavishly follow the politically correct line and perhaps also as someone who didn't know when to keep quiet for their own good. Foundation Status was tantalisingly close for UHMB and there is no doubt that senior management passionately believed that this had to be the correct direction of travel for the organisation and that pretty much any sacrifice was justifiable to preserve the future integrity of the Morecambe Bay NHS Trust. However, the senior management making such decisions did not have to see what was going on, day in and day out on the wards and in the theatres and A&E departments in order to try and drive this measure through. Furthermore, after some six to seven years as clinical lead, without any regular protected time and working 48+ clinical hours a week in addition to the lead work, on-call work and extra free evening and weekend sessions, I was exhausted and felt very stale. It was time for someone else to take over and I fervently hoped that I could be left to concentrate on my core clinical practice and perhaps spend a little more time with my family, now that Edward, Robert and William were all growing up rapidly.

One of my emails, sent to management on 10th May 2010, about the time that I was stepping down as clinical lead was as follows:

Subject: *Problems on ward 34*

Dear ...,

I'd like to pass on some concerns from this morning. I've mentioned on a number of occasions in the past my concerns about the pressures on staff on the surgical wards in the centenary building. It was the first thing that I mentioned to ... after her appointment, several years ago now.

Unfortunately, things have, if anything, worsened. I attended Ward 34 this morning intending to carry out a joint case with ... This was cancelled because of lack of beds. As there did not seem to be any other members of the urology team available to do a ward round I took it upon myself to stay on Ward 34 and see the urology inpatients here and on Wards 33 and 37.

*My understanding is that there were **45** medical outliers in surgical beds this morning. Ward 34 was given a list of 11 surgical patients requiring admission for today's operating lists. Needless to say, they were full, and were also two nursing staff down as well as missing two FY1 [junior] doctors. In short, it was a dangerous shambles. At one stage I was informed that patients were being taken to theatre without any bed to go into postoperatively. In the midst of all of this a group of medical students turned up expecting to be taught!*

I have spent the morning going round and sorting out the problems at consultant level as best I can. Having done the consultant ward round I have then started again and done an FY1 level ward round, writing in notes, filling in request forms, taking urgent imaging requests down to x-ray etc. and at other stages helping the hard-pressed nursing staff to pick up a patient who had fallen over, helping a patient to get dressed and wiping the bottom of another patient who had been faecally incontinent. It's really important to point out that no one was slacking on the ward, there simply were not enough staff to work under the pressure that was being exerted this morning.

It really concerns me to see just how dangerously overstretched the wards are at present. The danger is magnified by the absolute obsession with pushing elective cases through at all cost which results in the sickest inpatients being neglected in order to deal with each new influx of cases for theatre. The situation is compounded again in urology by the habit of withdrawing people from their scheduled ward rounds in order to cover other elective activities. It has reached a stage where I would not wish one of my relatives to be treated at the RLI.

I hope that this e-mail does not cause offence, but I suspect that middle and senior management have little knowledge of the gritty reality of what is going on on the wards. We are all aware of the adverse publicity attracted by Trusts elsewhere who neglected their most vulnerable patients in an all-out drive to attain Foundation Status. I would hate to see Morecambe Bay fall into the same trap.

Another email to management from that time is as follows:

Dear ...,

I ought to bring to your attention yesterday's events at the RLI. We had 7 patients on an all-day inpatient list. There were no beds (as usual) and the day turned into a dangerous and indefensible shambles, with multiple delays, numerous list changes, two patients being operated on having been allocated beds, only for the beds to be withdrawn during surgery resulting in them having to be held in recovery. It is only a matter of time until someone makes a major mistake as a result of this kind of chaos.

I asked that two of the afternoon patients were cancelled when it became clear that we couldn't do two of the morning patients because of bed shortages. This was ignored and the afternoon patients were brought in anyway. Although the anaesthetist and theatre staff were good enough to stay late and we worked on until nearly 6.30pm, we still didn't finish the list and I think that we treated the patients appallingly. I'm told that yesterday's routine admissions went ahead despite the fact that the police had been called during the night to placate patients being held in up to 9 ambulances due to lack of A&E capacity and when I finally went home last night we had minus 12 beds in the RLI.

Finally, I was really shocked to find out that a female patient had been held in the 'recovery 2' bay at the RLI for 48 hours, since Sunday. Despite this, we continued to admit non-cancer and non-urgent cases whilst denying this sick lady a ward bed of her own. How can this possibly be defended, and how does this fit with our Trust motto?

Our Trust motto at the time was 'The needs of our patients will drive everything we do' and tensions were high in the organisation. The Board was struggling for survival and whilst the consultant body mostly seemed to believe that the Board had taken a wrong turn, management in general sided with the executive. I'd undoubtedly declared my own loyalties by speaking out publicly against the Trust's direction at one of the big Trust meetings held in Grange-Over-Sands, held precisely because of the clinical concerns of the workforce. These took place at the large and impressive Netherwood Hotel and were attended by consultants and senior managers from all three sites across the Trust. Indeed, at the first meeting to discuss the issues over Foundation Status I was the first consultant on my feet to express concerns about clinical standards, safety and the direction of the Trust once the discussion was opened up to questions from the attendees.

Another email to management from me in July 2010 read:

I was supposed to be at WGH today, helping … and …
… is in clinic at QVH (Morecambe). We have an acutely bleeding patient on ward 37 that I am about to take to theatre and no one to sort out the rest of the acutely ill patients at RLI. Tomorrow will be even worse, with no middle grade again and all the other consultants 45 miles away on the other side of the Bay.

This is all terribly dangerous and, as I've pointed out on numerous occasions, we need to drop the obsession with keeping elective activities going at the expense of our most vulnerable sick in-patients. We cannot rely on our middle grades as their general surgical activities/leave/compensatory rest means that they are unavailable most of the time, and we need to get used to the idea of taking elective activities down for safety's sake when … is unavaila-

ble, rather than playing dice with the lives of our most needy patients for the sake of hitting targets.

I had more than one comment from fellow colleagues that my attitude had been noted by senior management and that I was considered to be rocking the boat. I had accompanying warnings about the hazards of speaking out under these circumstances and, on registering my deep unhappiness by stepping down as clinical lead, I was immediately punished with a 10% pay cut.

This was very unfair. Losing my clinical lead supplement pay was obviously reasonable. However, I'd never been given a pay rise to reflect the extra time spent on the clinical lead post, even when doubling up and being clinical lead for North Cumbria too. Nor were there any dedicated sessions for clinical lead work that would now become free time. Hence there was no justification for a further cut on top of losing the clinical lead supplement. Despite my protestations the Surgical Division pushed the cut through anyway and I suddenly found myself a good £1000 a month worse off, on top of losing the clinical lead allowance.

My new unpopularity with management was brought home to me with a vengeance early in 2011.

Just before Christmas 2010 my father suddenly died. He'd continued to work into his 70's as a pharmacist (receiving a letter from the President of the Royal Pharmaceutical Society, congratulating him on fifty years unbroken service to the public), before suffering at least two strokes. Admitted to the Royal Preston Hospital at the end of 2010 with diarrhoea and dehydration, he'd seemed well when we'd visited a couple of days earlier, smiling and interacting with the boys. We had no warning of the shrill 1.30am phone call that came through, the morning of the 23rd December, just before Christmas, telling us that he was critically ill and to come at once.

By the time the family and I got to the ward my father had just passed away. I managed just a few private moments of goodbye with his cold and waxy looking body before having to turn my back and walk away for the last time. The nursing staff were clearly busy and anxious to prepare the body for the mortuary.

This all sounds desperately upsetting and sad, but I can't honestly say that I felt desperately distressed. Although the body was clearly that of my father, he looked very dignified and very much at peace after several years of suffering. My memories, extending back through the previous nearly half-century of laughter, love and good, wise advice were so different from those last few moments with him that I couldn't help but feel a sense of relief alongside the inevitable crushing loss. His long struggle with ageing and frailty was over.

Looking back, I remember hoping that I had lived up to my father's plans and aspirations for me. I couldn't have asked for two better and more supportive parents and in turn I was determined to do justice to him by delivering the eulogy at his funeral. Never a good public speaker, I was nevertheless clear that this ought to be my final duty and tribute.

The NHS, however, had other ideas and it was at this point that my stance on the Trust's bid for Foundation Status again seemed to come back to bite me.

I worked through Christmas and Boxing Day without compassionate leave, having been timetabled to be on-call for both, as well as New Year's Eve on-call. After all, I reasoned, why spoil someone else's festive season by requesting compassionate leave when my own was a write off anyway? It wasn't easy and I remember struggling to try and stay composed and to concentrate on what the nursing staff were saying during the Christmas Day and Boxing Day ward rounds. However, once Christmas was out of the way I phoned the surgical divisional offices to ask for a half day off as compassionate leave to attend the funeral.

I was bluntly turned down on the basis that the half day in question was a clinic. The clinic in question was not just full but overbooked, and the Trust couldn't afford to miss targets by having a clinic full of Guaranteed Activity Date (GAD) patients (a political target) put back. I was also told that I hadn't given a minimum of six weeks' notice, as was standard when booking leave.

I don't usually struggle to keep my temper under control, but this was a major test. In the end, I managed to keep my cool and simply told the anonymous female manager on the other end of the phone that she was very welcome to bring the patients in as usual, but there was only one place that I was going to be on that particular half day, and that wasn't in a urological surgery clinic. In the end and after some mutterings which involved a second female voice, she relented (partially) saying that she'd arrange for the clinic to be moved to my next free half-day off. In the end there was no compassionate leave and it was abundantly clear that management were not, from this point on, going to make my life easy.

Worse was to come as, just two to three weeks later, several newspapers ran stories on me, ranging from the Sun's 'Teenager loses testicle in cancer bungle' to the Mail's 'Teenager has testicle removed after diagnosed with cancer... then he is told: *It was just a cyst.*'

I never managed to find out how these stories got into the national media. They related to a case from around a year earlier that had featured in the Cumbria newspaper, the North West Evening Mail and where I'd been accused of misdiagnosing a testicular cancer. However, I was assured by the Trust's media office that the stories had not been passed on either by the patient himself or the local paper, coming instead from a news agency in the Midlands.

The patient in question had indeed been provisionally given a diagnosis of testicular cancer and, after urgent surgery, the lump in question had been found to be an epidermoid cyst (identical-looking to a cancer on scanning and not to be muddled with an epididymal cyst, which is always benign in practice).

Thankfully, I'd told the patient (as well as carefully documenting it) that there was a 5% chance of the lump being benign. However, this didn't stop a series of lurid headlines, which were then picked up by the internet and spread across blogs, news websites and medical negligence websites across several continents.

Two weeks later, I absent-mindedly opened an innocent looking letter from the General Medical Council (GMC). It looked just like something announcing that my subscriptions had gone up (again) but the contents had me instantly leaning over the kitchen sink, retching. It was a notification that I was now subject to a top level 'Stream one' GMC enquiry on account of the media articles. Suddenly, there was a real possibility that I could be publicly hauled before the GMC and struck off, never practising again.

The rest of 2011 and on into 2012 was not a happy time. I felt unsupported and very alone. The Trust made no effort to get the media stories taken down, nor to offer me any support over the GMC enquiry. Particularly coming so soon after my father's untimely death and lack of compassionate leave and with the ongoing 10% pay cut, it suddenly seemed as though everything was going very wrong.

The months afterwards passed in a blur of anxiety and distraction, with barely a waking hour passing when I wasn't reminded in some way of the threat hanging over my vocation. It was well after the summer (including a spoiled summer holiday) before the GMC dropped the action against me, telling me that I had no case to answer. Nearly a year on, I finally extracted an apology from some of the tabloid press.

> *An article in Sun Online on 19th January 2011: 'Testicle removed in cancer bungle' referred to Mr Peter Duffy, a consultant urologist, employed by University Hospitals of Morecambe Bay NHS Trust. We did not intend to suggest by our headline or our interpretation of events that Mr Duffy had negligently carried out his duties as the consultant involved.*
>
> *The GMC has since ruled beyond doubt that Mr Duffy behaved professionally and appropriately to the required standards at all times.*
>
> *We apologise to Mr Duffy for any embarrassment.*

During this period it was very clear that the organisations giving me the greatest support were my private insurer and the local private hospital, even though this was an exclusively NHS issue.

After my actions had been fully vindicated (the expert witness for the GMC praised my actions as being fully in accordance with best practice) I pursued the GMC for an answer as to why I had been investigated in the first place. In a phone call to me a senior GMC manager implied that the original story and complaint had almost certainly come from within the Trust and I recalled that the local newspaper, the Lancaster Guardian had also been tipped off. Thankfully they chose not to publish.

I CONTINUED TO WORK hard after my father's death. The job seemed to be getting more and more demanding and I appeared to be picking up an ever increasing amount of emergency work. I would be in the hospital several evenings per week, even to the point where one of the regular theatre nurses on the evening shift at the RLI asked me if I was the only urological surgeon that ever did emergency on-call work. It was difficult and over this dark and depressing period I struggled to cope with the pressure of day to day NHS work whilst trying to reconcile myself with my father's death and simultaneously coping with the tabloid headlines, GMC enquiry and my ongoing 10% pay cut. It seemed clear to me that, in addition to the phone call warning me about Mr Madhra's intentions, I had made enemies in management as a consequence of my speaking out against low clinical standards and as a result of the comparisons that I had made with Mid Staffs. As I struggled on and particularly with the benefit of hindsight, it now seems inevitable that my health would take a serious knock.

THIS CAME IN 2012, some six months after the GMC had exonerated me and shortly after the tabloids had published their apologies.

I began a weekend on-call in mid to late April 2012 after a week when other colleagues had been timetabled to be on-call, dealing with the emergencies. As described in my Employment Tribunal witness statement several years later, I carried out a ward round on the Saturday morning and before I had even finished on the first of several wards on the extended ward round, I had booked four patients for emergency operations. All of them should, in my own opinion have been operated on at least a day earlier and three of the four had been waiting for several days. My description of that day was provided to the Employment Tribunal some six years later as follows:

I was admitted to the CCU [the Cardiac Ward] *on 30th April 2012 and if my recollection is correct then it was one or two weekends before this that the four cases occurred.*

The first was a young girl who had been admitted under the general surgeons, I think with suspected appendicitis. She continued running temperatures post-operatively with raised septic markers and subsequently was found on ultrasound scanning to have a hydronephrotic [blocked] *kidney. When I came on duty on the Saturday morning she was being conservatively managed with antibiotics alone with no plan for emergency drainage of her suspected infected obstructed kidney.*

The second case was one of our own ICU nurses, came in midweek with severe left upper quadrant pain after sneezing. She had a ruptured, hydronephrotic kidney with retro-peritoneal urine leakage and was septic with an E. Coli [bacterial] *infection in her urine. Again, her ongoing retro-peritoneal leakage of infected urine from a ruptured infected kidney was being managed with antibiotics alone.*

The third case was an elderly Italian gentleman with locally advanced and hormone resistant prostate cancer who had come in with a blocked stent and with an ultrasound report clearly stating that the 'previously atrophic and stented kidney is now hydronephrotic'. He had been having rigors [high temperatures] *and had ESBL* [a highly antibiotic-resistant bug] *in his urine. He was being treated with antibiotics and a referral to the microbiology team with no plan to change his blocked stent and drain his infected obstructed kidney (very similar to the Mr A. avoidable death).*

Finally, I also inherited an elderly man in his 80's who had rising septic markers, dramatically deteriorating renal function and bilateral hydronephrosis on US, again being treated with antibiotics alone. I organised a CT [computerised body scan] *scan on him (expecting to find some retro-peritoneal pathology). In fact he had bilateral obstructing stones with one of the kidneys infected too.*

All the cases had sufficient information to make the diagnosis of some variant of infected obstructed kidney at least one to two days earlier. My recollection is that Mr Jain was on-call for the week leading up to that weekend. The case details ought to be available on ORMIS [Operating Room Management Information System] *as I operated on them all later that same Saturday (after a very long and complex ward round sorting out other issues and a call out to Barrow too, acquiring my cardiac issues in the process)! It should not take too much work to find out the exact details.*

Having completed my rounds of the urology patients in the RLI, I had hoped to start operating on all four emergency cases in the afternoon. However, I got called out to FGH for a sick patient who was septic after a set of prostate biopsies. The journey to FGH from Lancaster is a 2½ hour round trip and, having got back to Lancaster at around 6pm, I only finished the final operation at about midnight. I had nothing to eat during the day, surviving on cups of coffee. Unsurprisingly, it was at this point that the strains of the last eighteen months of excessive workload, bereavement, GMC enquiries and newspaper headlines caught up with me.

I started getting extra heart beats, called ventricular ectopics or ventricular extra-systoles. These are extra, premature heartbeats and, as they are not co-ordinated, the heart doesn't beat properly. Worse, the heart then pauses, as though it is re-booting itself before resuming its normal rhythm. It's pretty alarming, especially the compensatory pause and you find yourself holding your breath, waiting to see if it really will restart! At the time, I only knew that my heart rhythm kept becoming irregular and that I started feeling faint from time-to-time with odd thumps and knocks from within my chest and then a pause before my heart kicked back into its normal rhythm.

On Monday the 30th August I offered to cover an operating list for Carl Rowbotham at Lancaster. Still suffering from regular ectopic heartbeats I should, in hindsight, have cancelled the list and taken some time off. However, we're all aware of the disruption that this causes to the patients and their families and I wrongly made the decision to press on and try to work through the day.

The operating list was nothing short of a disaster. My ectopic heart beats became much more rapid during my first operation of the day; a prostate resection (TURP). The anaesthetist suddenly realised that I wasn't well, commenting 'OMG Peter, you've gone the most peculiar colour.... Are you OK?!'

No one was available to relieve me and I managed to struggle through, being utterly soaked in sweat by the end, my theatre 'blues' appearing black as they were wet through with perspiration and my surgical gloves hanging off me like scalded skin as a result of all the sweat that had run down my arms and into the surgical gloves. My hands were shaking so much that I had to get the nurse assisting me to hold them still whilst I put the patient's catheter in at the end of the procedure. The anaesthetist and theatre matron instructed me to sit down and put my head between my knees whilst they got the patient off the operating table. I ended up in the resuscitation area of the Emergency Department before being admitted to the coronary care unit (CCU).

Mercifully my ectopic heartbeats reduced significantly on the CCU once I was given beta-blockers and oxygen and thankfully the blood tests suggested that I hadn't had a myocardial infarction or heart attack as everyone feared, although I had to stay in until the early hours of the morning to find this out. I was discharged home way after midnight that night and had about three months off sick.

I actually recovered very quickly once out of the hospital atmosphere, being out jogging within a couple of weeks of my admission. The main delay was that I had to wait for a CT coronary angiogram (a scan of the heart arteries) at Blackpool Victoria Hospital which had a three month wait (despite me ringing most days to ask if there were any short-notice cancellations), before I was allowed back to work in the NHS. In the meantime, I occupied myself with trying to get fit again and, once fully recovered, carried out some limited private work as part of a phased return to work and after making sure that I'd secured permission from Belinda, my NHS line manager.

At the time, this seemed sensible, but I was clearly being watched with hostile intent at this point by Mr Jain, and this decision was something else that would come back to cause me trouble, several years later.

My return to work meeting was held on the 13th July 2012 and I met with Belinda and Lesley from HR (Human Resources). Both were sympathetic, sensible and understanding. Amongst other things that we talked about, I mentioned the large excess of emergency workload that I seemed to be carrying and the perception (amongst the theatre and anaesthetic staff as well as myself) that there might not be the same commitment to emergency work amongst some of my other colleagues in the department. In the end, as I felt that I'd been left quite a number of improperly managed patients to sort out prior to my cardiac episode and since this was far from the first time that this had happened, we agreed to ask for an independent audit of my emergency workload, carried out by the head of theatres.

The audit retrospectively covered the previous year and the results were utterly astonishing. I'd suspected that I might be carrying out rather more surgery than some of my contemporaries, but no one dreamed that the differences would be this stark. I was clearly being left huge amounts of emergency work to do, something between a third and a half of all the emergencies in the department.

Duffy – 50 cases
Mr A – 22
Mr B – 17
Mr C – 14
Mr D – 13
Mr E – 7

It was clear that these results needed to be urgently communicated back to the department. At the time, we had an on-call system where we were all in turn responsible for sorting out all the emergencies in our on-call session, passing anything that hadn't been dealt with to the next on-call consultant. Normally, this system ought to even out the workload, as, on average, the on-call consultant might pass on the occasional case that he or she hadn't managed to deal with, but would also inherit a similar number. These results were indicative of a major imbalance in the workload and suggested that not everyone was pulling their weight in getting all of their emergencies done during their shift.

It was agreed that I would present the results at one of our departmental meetings. I was very nervous and recall my voice trembling, shaking and breaking as I spoke about the results of the theatre emergency audit. I feared that these figures would not be well received and this was certainly the case. Mr Jain and Mr Naseem both joined together to accuse me of harming patients by operating on them when they didn't need surgery and of obstructing their access to the emergency theatre. It was further claimed that the NHS theatre staff obstructed both of these individuals from being able to fulfil their share of the emergency work and there clearly wasn't going to be a low key, careful, mature and informed discussion and analysis of these results. I was completely tongue-tied by the ferocity of the attack on me, my voice began shaking and I hastily backed off and dropped the subject. It wasn't revisited again for at least a couple of years.

As well as my concerns about emergency cover, I also continued to express my concerns about clinical standards in general, within the urology department at the RLI but also other hospitals within the Morecambe Bay Trust during my return to work meeting. I summarised my concerns in a letter sent to Belinda and Lesley after the return-to-work meeting was over.

> *There can be no doubt that a greater emphasis on targets and efficiency has brought down waiting times and improved treatment for a lot of patients. However, I feel very strongly that we have become far too obsessed as an organisation with such issues and have lost touch with our primary function; namely to provide high quality, safe and consistent care for <u>all</u> our patients, not just those who happen to advance UHMB's cause financially or with respect to targets. We discussed the common practice of keeping sick patients waiting on trolleys in A&E whilst continuing to admit routine cases for elective surgery, and the practice of leaving sick patients requiring emergency surgery on wards for sometimes days at a time before they can receive their emergency surgery, whilst*

pressing on with elective admissions for sometimes genuinely trivial conditions. I've certainly had patients who've been left in agony and have been starved for three days before they've been able to get their emergency surgery. If we treated animals that way, there'd be outrage. I'm sure that you will understand the very significant extra strain and unhappiness that results from working under such conditions, particularly when treating patients in such a fashion clearly breaches the GMC's code of professional behaviour.

I went on to say:

As we discussed, I believe that the 'equity' of emergency work has played a role in the overshoot. I don't want to personalise this, but I do firmly believe that some people in the department will do everything possible to sort out emergencies on their shift, whilst others are content to push much less hard and pass outstanding work on to the next on-call consultant. This obviously creates an imbalance and distorts the workload around the department.

These concerns continued into 2013 when I sent an email to the chief executive Ms Daniel in March about standards. It was dated 13th March and I received no response.

Dear Ms Daniel,

I'm not sure how much feedback you get from the front-line, but I feel that I ought to let you know just how dangerous yesterday's all day urology list felt. Having always enjoyed operating, I now dread my all day alternate Tuesdays at the RLI. We are always short of beds, equipment and experienced staff and it has got to the stage where I sleep very poorly on a Monday night before such a list and even more poorly afterwards.

Yesterday was even more stressful and dangerous than usual. I skipped breakfast to get in early and started the day at 7.40am with an admissions lounge full of patients and staff, all milling about. No cubicles available so I ended up consenting three of the four morning patients in the staff room. No notes for one elderly unfit lady with bladder cancer and only one male bed. We finally got the list underway and managed to do three of the mornings four cases, having changed the order of the list several times to account for changes in bed availability. We had a major equipment breakdown mid-morning with one of our ageing resectoscopes refusing to work and finally being noted to be sparking internally and overheating (very dangerous) and were finally informed after 12.00 and with our third patient still underway that we had a bed for our last patient (the list finishes at 12.30). The latter patient then had to be added on to the four afternoon patients who had meantime been admitted to the admissions lounge despite the lack of beds. We were then left with five patients to do in the afternoon.

I went back to the admissions lounge to apologise and explain to the 80 year old lady and her daughter, (who had been kept starved and waiting all morning) and the mornings experience in the admissions lounge was then repeated with no time for lunch. We then faced a mad scramble through the afternoon list to try and get the five cases done. All day, we faced a lack of equipment (kit supposedly prioritised by CSSD hadn't been prioritised), extra kit being sent from Kendal arrived late, turnover between patients was slow due to lack of staff, the Lorenzo op note and discharge summary computer repeatedly crashed, and on at least two occasions, pasted op' details from the last-but-one patient into the discharge summary of the last patient (very dangerous again) and our electronic op/discharge summary/theatre rebooking/MDT [multi-disciplinary team] booking work has expanded to the point where it cannot safely be done in the gap between operations, especially where we're rushing to compensate for lack of beds, meaning that I'm still frantically typing whilst the next patient is going on the table.

I finally staggered out of the hospital just before 7 pm. I can honestly say that during my third of a century in healthcare incorporating at various stages 1:2 rotas, 140 hour weeks and 50+ hours without sleep, I've never felt so dangerous to my patients as I felt yesterday. I couldn't sleep last night as every time I drifted off, I had nightmares about the day, and particularly nightmares about operating on the wrong patient.

I really hope we can do something to make this organisation safer.

I hope that you don't mind my contacting you directly, but I feel that often the day-to-day issues never get fed up to the more senior levels within the organisation.

Yours sincerely,

There was no reply and a further similar letter went in about clinical standards from an anaesthetic colleague and myself in September 2013. Once again, there was no reply or acknowledgement.

As well as my concerns about standards in general in UHMB I continued to express my concerns about standards in the urology department. At a departmental meeting in mid-2013 I again spoke up about a female patient who had been left on the ward passing large volumes of blood and clots in her urine for around a fortnight without surgical attention, simply being handed on from consultant to consultant and being managed with only repeated blood transfusions and catheter changes. Luckily, an attentive junior doctor brought her to my attention after about two weeks of sitting on the ward haemorrhaging and a subsequent cystoscopy (bladder inspection under general anaesthetic) 24 hours later by myself revealed a bladder cancer. Having been able to remove this at the same operation, she immediately stopped bleeding and was discharged home within 24 to 48 hours.

However, things could have ended very differently indeed and she should in my opinion have been taken to theatre for emergency surgery at least seven days earlier. Once again I was very nervous about presenting her case and once again my concerns triggered another furious exchange of views between some colleagues, with each declining to accept any responsibility and blaming someone else. I again dropped the subject, but it seemed clear that expressing low key and off the record verbal concerns was not going to change standards for the better. For the first time I formally expressed concerns to the Clinical Director in my annual NHS appraisal from 2012-14, where I stated:

I do not have full confidence in the commitment to the on-call service exhibited by some of my colleagues. A case occurred just a month or so ago in where I organised an urgent diagnostic bladder tumour resection for a patient with large volume metastatic bladder cancer [cancer that has widely spread], *as first patient on the emergency list at the behest of the MDT meeting. A histological diagnosis was vital for the patient to receive prompt chemotherapy. I was prepared to stay late and do the case, even though not on-call, but a colleague arrived and sent me home, saying that he was on-call and would make sure that case was done. I received a call later that evening, saying that the case had been cancelled by my col-league and the patient sent home. He has still to start his chemotherapy now, some two months on. I therefore believe firmly in taking ownership and responsibility for my patients and make no apology for my commitment to seeing their care through to a satis-factory conclusion.*

In late 2013, relationships within the department took another downturn with a spoiled half term holiday. I'd had a previous issue over a family holiday being blocked, the colleague in question only agreeing to allow me to take the holiday after he'd secured a 'trade-off' where I'd had to agree to work his Christmas on-call for him. On this occasion, just days before the planned holiday, I found out that the same colleague had booked up an extra operating list on the weekend that I'd asked him to swap. As he was now unavailable, I was informed by a senior divisional manager that I was required to commit to paying for a locum consultant for the first Saturday of the holiday (potentially a four figure sum) in order to get away on time.

Officially the explanation for all of this was a 'misunderstanding' but I was quietly informed afterwards and off-the-record that the intention all along was to 'teach you a lesson.'

I returned home exhausted and sleep deprived after a thoroughly spoiled holiday, fully expecting a four figure bill and rather predicta-bly suffered another recurrence of my cardiac rhythm problems when I was once again sent home by the theatre matron and anaesthetist, after yet again nearly passing out during an operation in a near-identical re-run of my previous heart issues.

Occupational health signed me off until after the New Year with a recurrence of stress related ventricular ectopics. My stress levels were judged by the occupational health consultant to be *nearly off the scale* but I still wanted to work and be of use to the department, even though I was not judged fit to do clinical work.

As a result of discussions with Belinda my line manager I undertook to carry out a 'validation exercise', going through the notes of patients who were on our very excessive waiting list for outpatient appointments and writing to any which I felt were unnecessary, discharging them back to the GP.

At the time we had a huge backlog of what are called 'follow-up' outpatient appointments. These are patients who don't need admission but are being seen and 'followed up' in the outpatients department for things like prostate cancer, cystitis, kidney stones etc. Because of the huge backlog of work, the Trust had to lay on extra clinics, known as AAS (additional activity session) clinics, carried out either in consultant's spare or free time, evenings or weekends.

There was concern (well justified as it turned out) that not everyone being brought back was really needing outpatient follow-up. Perhaps the premium-rate or overtime 'waiting list initiative' AAS clinics, remunerated at the standard rate of £500 per half day session were in themselves encouraging some clinicians to 'recirculate' patients who could otherwise be discharged? In doing so, the waits for clinics would remain excessive, breaching the Government's targets for waiting times and thus keeping the demand for premium rate clinics high. In turn, managers would then be obliged to put on more premium rate clinics in order to avoid missing the NHS waiting time targets.

The validation work began in late 2013 and it rapidly became very clear indeed to both me and to Belinda that there was a huge amount of unnecessary work going on in the department. Patients who had been sent in for investigation by their GP and had completed all their tests were being brought back for follow-up appointments time after time, many of them having entirely negative tests and most having no significant ongoing illness to justify their follow-up. Even patients who had failed to show up were being repeatedly rebooked back for further appointments. Many of these follow up appointments were happening in the £500/session additional AAS clinics.

I forwarded on numerous examples of these inappropriate follow-up appointments to management and set about reviewing and discharging the patients. It is a measure of the sheer amount of unnecessary work that we were getting through about 40-60 extra AAS clinics every month, just within the urology department alone, perhaps 700-800 patients (up to £30,000 worth of unnecessary extra overtime each month). Incredibly and equipped with no more than a desktop computer and access to the patients' records and results, I was able to go through these patients records and discharge up to 50% of them simply by reviewing their notes and results. Some of this work was done during my sick leave but I voluntarily continued with it after my return to work, carrying out the notes reviews from the urology office during my evenings and weekends. Perhaps unsurprisingly, these efforts did not meet with universal approval, several colleagues who were making considerable amounts of money from the extra AAS clinics being considerably less than impressed and making their unhappiness over this exercise very clear.

An example of unnecessary follow-up is below, with an introductory email from myself, followed by the actual letter from the female patient's appointment, both of these having been presented as evidence to my Employment Tribunal hearing. The letter makes it clear that she had no symptoms, her infections had resolved and all her tests had proved negative. Yet she was going to be brought back to the clinic again in a few months. It is worth noting that the clinic in question was an AAS clinic, would have started at about 5–5.30pm and should have lasted at least 3.5 hours:

From: Duffy Peter
Sent: x April 2014 07:15
To: ...;(UHMB) ...;(UHMB)
Subject
Importance: High

... &...,

I stayed late last night and got in very early again this am to try and keep up with the validations. PLEASE take a look at the below. It is typical of the kind of frankly unprofessional and probably fraudulent behaviour that is going on in some parts of the department. ...'s evening clinic last night, for which he'll probably bill you £500, finished at 7.20pm. I think he saw about 10–11 patients. I suspect he contributed little or nothing, judging from the sort of patients that he's recirculating and I'm finding in this validation exercise. Isn't this terribly wrong that he's ripping the Trust and department off quite blatantly whilst I'm spending my weekends, evenings and early mornings trying to repair the damage and discharge these patients by letter for free......

Very, very unhappy Peter.

Here is the consultant's letter to the GP:

Many thanks for referring Mrs. ... with a history of urinary tract infections, but currently she is totally asymptomatic and has got no urinary trouble at all.

In the past she has had appendicectomy and hysterectomy performed. Currently she is on amilodipine for hypertension.

On examination, she is good for her age. Abdominal examination was otherwise unremarkable.

Dipstick performed in out-patients today showed no evidence of blood, nitrates or protein in her urine.

An ultrasound scan performed by yourself showed normal kidneys and bladder.

As she is asymptomatic, no further action is required. However, I will keep an eye on her for the time being. I have given her a review appointment to see me again in 4 months' time.

Yours sincerely,

The sorts of numbers involved and percentages being discharged are revealed in the email below.

From Duffy Peter
Sent 28 January 2014 11.48
To ...;(UHMB) ...;(UHMB)
Subject: Validations 17th Jan..xlsx URGENT PLEASE

Latest validations: 300 done now and 203 provisionally dis-
charged.
Pls could you send me on some more. I've only 9 to do (will
prob try and finish this evening) and then I've run out.

The validation work continued from late 2013 right through until my last days in the Trust in mid to late 2016. It is difficult to know exactly how many patients I ultimately discharged, with the Trust denying any knowledge of the exercise to the 2018 Employment Tribunal. However, just a brief skim through my Trust laptop before handing it back revealed the RTX numbers (unique patient numbers to Morecambe Bay) of over 2,000 patients with somewhere between 25 and 50% of these being written to and discharged. Such patients were often being recirculated several times, with clinics having perhaps 12-14 patients in them. Each clinic was probably costing the Trust well in excess of £1,000 once the overtime costs of nursing staff, secretarial time, receptionists etc. had been factored in. With many hundreds, probably thousands of patients having been discharged, it seems likely that Belinda's and my efforts saved Morecambe Bay's Critical Care Division a substantial six figure sum.

It is utterly surreal to reflect on the fact that, having benefited so much from the exercise it was management within this very same Critical Care Division that was to ultimately and entirely falsely accuse me of fraudulent behaviour and wasting six-figure sums and was to be the main architect of my unfair constructive dismissal some 3½ years later.

CHAPTER NINE

Snide and prejudice

ON THE 14TH DECEMBER 2013 I was nearly three years on from my father's untimely death. I was still off sick after the spoiled holiday and was concentrating on trying to regain my grip on a job that I'd always felt to be an absolute vocation but which seemed to be being increasingly forced from my grasp. Luxuriously fast asleep for an hour or two, having consumed another of Fiona's excellent roast meals as well as a couple of generous glasses of wine, I was rudely jerked awake at perhaps 11.30pm with an emergency call from the BMI Hospital (the local private hospital). They had a surgical crisis; an NHS patient who had had an orthopaedic (joint) operation now couldn't pass urine. The on-call resident doctor couldn't manage to pass a catheter to relieve the patient who was now in very significant pain.

I pointed out the fact that I had been asleep, was signed off sick and explicitly wasn't supposed to be performing any emergency procedures, had consumed alcohol and wasn't on-call; it was Mr Jain who was on-call for the night. The nurse profusely apologised and hung up.

Unable to sleep after the call, I got up, waited for the palpitations to settle, made myself a hot drink and having failed to get back to sleep, phoned the hospital back to check that the situation had been resolved. The phone was answered with a comment along the lines of 'Thank God you've phoned back,' from the on-duty nurse. I was aghast to be informed that Mr Jain had refused to attend, declaring that he was 90 miles away and had instructed that the patient be transferred to the Acute Surgical Unit at the RLI. They in turn had refused to accept the patient as the on-call consultant (Mr Jain) had just admitted that he was 90 miles away and therefore unavailable. The nurse and patient felt 'abandoned' and the patient was now in agony (try to imagine what it's like having your bladder really really painfully full, continuing to fill and being unable to pee despite your best efforts...).

This left me in an impossible position, particularly as it was the night of the departmental Christmas party and everyone else who might have been able to help was at the party a good few miles away, not on-call and probably rather worse for wear. In the end, I had to make a snap decision. I asked the nurse to check that the patient was prepared to consent to me coming in and performing the procedure under such circumstances. Unsurprisingly he agreed with alacrity. Unsure if I might be just over the limit, I jogged to the BMI Hospital, about half a mile away, passing the RLI on the way and picking up the kit to carry out a suprapubic catheter insertion (a special kit to make an incision and insert a catheter drainage tube directly through the skin of the lower abdomen into the bladder). Mercifully for the patient (and for me under the circumstances) the procedure went smoothly and a huge jet of high-pressure urine was emitted from the catheter, rising at least 18 inches into the air (I have done more than enough of these to have remembered to step smartly aside at this point), immediately followed by a groan of relief from the patient.

This incident clearly should never have happened and, coming on top of the obvious in-balance in emergency work, this was the first time that I made a formal written complaint about a colleague since the mid-2000s. Although the incident ended happily, it could clearly have had a number of very different (and very unhappy) endings and could well have threatened my GMC registration again if I'd had a major surgical complication, operating whilst judged unfit to operate, off sick and under the influence of alcohol. However, Mr Jain clearly didn't see my point of view and made his anger over my complaint very clear to all. He openly treated me as a threat (which, in hindsight I suppose I was) and I always felt extremely uncomfortable in his company from this point on. In a taste of things to come, no one spoke to me about the investigation of the incident, or the conclusion and there was no feedback or change in practice whatsoever. The only noticeable difference was clearly the distinct worsening of Mr Jain's attitude towards me.

By now I had given up booking holidays and had told my line manager that I'd not be booking any more holiday time off and would simply work 52 weeks a year as I was too scared of further abuses of the annual leave system and the impact that this might have on my health. After quite a while without any annual leave, it was then agreed that Belinda would book my holidays and arrange cover to try and avoid a repetition of the previous holiday issues.

I had also given up using the shared consultant office and had moved out to work alongside the secretaries because of the atmosphere, the fear that I had of being cornered in there by one of my colleagues and the need to have witnesses around. I tried to avoid the main hospital entrance, entering and leaving by the back entrance by the staff canteen and accessing the urology departmental offices via the fire escape.

Departmental relationships continued to sour with email attacks on me by Mr Jain and Mr Naseem in early January 2014, much day-to-day personal hostility and with an anonymous email from Mr Jain in March 2014 which was passed on to me by a third party, the email and subsequent correspondence containing a series of accusations.

In May 2014 we had a truly huge clinical error by Mr Madhra. A patient turned up on the morning of his planned surgery, with the operation due to be carried out by myself, but listed to have the wrong kidney removed. I only picked up the error moments before the patient was due to be transferred up to the operating theatre for the operation.

As the patient was being seen by the anaesthetist at the time of my arrival for the operating list, I went to the notes and checked with the letter to the GP from the patient's last clinic appointment, which had been with Mr Madhra. This clearly stated that the patient had a left sided TCC (transitional cell carcinoma, a kind of cancer of the kidney lining and collecting tubes) and was to undergo a left nephroureterectomy (removal of the left kidney and ureter; the urine tube to the bladder). This is, of course, major irreversible surgery.

Alongside the letter to the GP was the booking form, filled in by hand and again specifying 'left radical nephroureterectomy'.

Thankfully, it has always been my practice to carefully cross reference the operation against not just the last letter, scan or X ray reports but against my own interpretation of them. Loading the images onto PACS (the NHS digital imaging system) I was immediately struck by how normal the left kidney looked. Turning to the patient's right kidney, it was this one that looked decidedly dodgy. With a sickening feeling I turned to the radiology consultant's report. This clearly stated *right* TCC.

The anaesthetist had now left, the patient was looking expectantly at me and the porters were already standing at the admissions lounge door waiting to take the patient to theatre.

Crunch time. Did I go with my own interpretation and the CT report, or with the theatre listing and last GP letter? Or did I confess to the patient that there was confusion over which kidney contained the cancer and which was the healthy one (in which case he'd probably and understandably have run screaming out of the nearest door). I made a snap decision to go with the former, mentally calculating that I'd have time to go through the notes again and double check whilst the patient went to sleep, as well as being able to double-check my own impressions with one of the consultant radiologists whilst the patient was being transferred up to theatre.

Thankfully after I'd consented the patient and he'd departed for the anaesthetic room, I found an earlier reference from Mr Cutting to suspicions of a right sided TCC and a consultant radiologist subsequently confirmed my impression that it was indeed the right kidney that was the problem one, the patient never realising how close to disaster he had been.

I arrived sweating profusely in the operating theatre just as the patient was being wheeled in from the anaesthetic room, gathered myself together, took some deep breaths, steadied my shaking fingers and proceeded to remove the right-sided kidney and ureter, immediately post-operatively declaring this as a major clinical incident which it clearly was. Had I gone ahead with the surgery as specified on the booking form and in the letter to the GP in the hospital notes, the patient would have had his healthy kidney removed and would have been left with the cancerous one which would then have had to be removed too, leaving him dependent on dialysis, an utter potential catastrophe (and one which had already happened once elsewhere in the NHS, making the national news).

My covering email stated:

This could easily have been a disaster attracting national media attention and ending my career had I carried out the procedure detailed in the original booking and referral.

I added, quoting from the NHS England Surgical Never Events Taskforce Report that:

No amount of World Health Organisation checklists, team briefings etc. will in themselves, prevent wrong site/side surgery if the original listing and referral is wrong, as any pre-op checklists are themselves predicated on the patient being correctly listed in the first place.

Whilst I was congratulated on my attention to detail, I also sensed a huge amount of resentment over my reporting of this incident. Yet after having repeatedly warned that we were making far too many basic and casual errors on far too many occasions, I really felt that I had no alternative, especially with the General Medical Council's unequivocal position on such errors: –

Doctors in particular have a duty to act when they believe patient's safety is at risk, or that patient's care or dignity is being compromised. Our guidance sets out our expectation that all doctors will, whatever their role, take appropriate action to raise and act on concerns about patient care, dignity and safety. As a doctor you must take prompt action if you think patient safety, dignity or comfort is being compromised.

Mr Madhra was subsequently suspended for the second time a couple of weeks later after yet another potentially catastrophic error, reported by a consultant colleague when he failed to act over a potential case of cord compression (another emergency requiring immediate action to minimise the risks of the patient being paralysed).

I had very much hoped that departmental standards might improve after such a major scare and near miss, my previous expressions of concern, the other potentially catastrophic near misses and the re-suspension of Mr Madhra. But within three months in August 2014 we had another near disaster, with a previously fit and healthy man being completely inexplicably sent home with a newly diagnosed but entirely untreated large and advanced bladder cancer, sepsis and renal (kidney) blockage and failure. The case was described in my evidence to the 2018 Employment Tribunal, reproduced from an earlier email:

> *The next case is a little difficult to pin down. It relates to a male patient who was (I think) in his early to mid-60's and who had presented with haematuria (blood in the urine) and a huge bladder mass, (I recall the CT scan showing a roughly 9-10cm bladder cancer). He also had bilaterally obstructed kidneys on imaging, grossly deranged renal function and raised septic markers* [both kidneys blocked and starting to fail with signs of incipient sepsis too].
>
> *I only came across him as I was called to the ward one evening (as the on-call urology consultant) to change his irrigating catheter to a two way one before his discharge home. I was appalled to see a clearly desperately unwell man (previously fit and healthy) who was being discharged home by Mr Jain and Mr Naseem with his management plan being re-admission on Mr Duffy's operating list in about 6 weeks for TURBT! I vividly recall phoning Carl Rowbotham and asking him if I'd died and been reincarnated into a parallel universe where we managed everything totally differently! I think that I saw him on a Thursday. There was no nephrostomy available* [an emergency kidney drain used in the X ray department under such circumstances] *and, having spoken to Professor Smith, consultant anaesthetist, we agreed to book him for*

an emergency TURBT and retrograde stenting [surgical removal of the bladder tumour and insertion of internal kidney drainage tubes] *on the Saturday morning to give us time to optimise him. If ... carries out an ORMIS search on Saturday TURBTs on the emergency list (there won't be many) then he'll find this patient. It was also a very prolonged resection taking all morning with bilateral retrograde stent insertion, so shouldn't take long to find. The procedure took place in the RLI and a clinical incident was definitely submitted. I recall Carl Rowbotham saying that I had no choice but to submit one.*

Unfortunately, the clinical error here involved both Mr Jain and Mr Naseem who had already made clear their deep resentment over the fact that I had reported Mr Madhra for listing the wrong kidney to be removed.

Once again, this was a terrible error of neglect. Bladder cancer can be a relatively innocuous entity in its earlier and least aggressive manifestations, but this cancer, 9 to 10cm in diameter, was clearly very advanced. Not only this but it was clearly invading through the bladder wall, blocking both kidneys and starting to cause kidney failure. On top of this, the patient's septic blood test markers were significantly raised, suggesting that at least one of the obstructed kidneys might be infected too. This could and should have been definitively dealt with days and days earlier.

I completed the procedure, spending the whole of what would otherwise have been a free Saturday morning on the case, resecting (removing) all the visible tumour, uncovering the blocked ureters and managing to get ureteric stents (drainage tubes) into both kidneys. Having already reported the previous case of the patient being listed for removal of the wrong kidney, this seemed to be a mistake of a similar magnitude to that made by Mr Madhra. I had no choice but to post-operatively submit the mandatory and inevitable clinical incident form.

I was phoned back a day or two after I had submitted the incident forms to warn me that both individuals were furious and utterly committed to revenge.

Once again I received no feedback from the investigations into either this case or the case of the patient being listed for removal of the wrong kidney.

This was followed by another inexcusable and inexplicable error in September 2014 by Mr Jain when a young, sexually naive teenager of about 16 presented with severe and acute testicular pain. Inexplicably, he was sent home on antibiotics for a sexually transmitted disease despite it being clearly recorded in the notes that he was a virgin (it is worth pointing out that, despite the regular trotting-out of excuses about public toilet seats, you cannot get a sexually transmitted infection without having some form of sex!). The correct and in my opinion barn-door obvious diagnosis was a testicular torsion, a surgical emergency where the testicle twists and cuts off its blood supply. The young man subsequently lost his testicle as a consequence of the inaction. I submitted a clinical incident about this too, after spending what should have been an afternoon off performing emergency surgery on the unfortunate young man to remove his necrotic, gangrenous testicle. Within a month (13th October 2014) there were in my opinion two further safety-critical errors. A frail, elderly man with an infected obstructed kidney and candidal sepsis (a fungal and very serious blood infection probably originating from the blocked kidney) was turned down for emergency surgery by Mr Jain, being deferred for the next consultant to sort out the following day. This was whilst another young man at Barrow who had presented with a priapism that same evening (an erection that won't go down) was sent back to his home from Furness General Hospital and instructed to get a taxi down to the Royal Lancaster Infirmary the following day.

Both of these were surgical emergencies. The recommendation from the Royal College of Surgeons for the treatment of infected obstructed kidneys is intervention within three hours, whilst priapism is an immediate emergency, as undue delay can result in the patient being left impotent (as I believe happened in this case). Having been left untreated from the previous evening, both cases were dealt with surgically by me the following day, even though I wasn't on-call and both were formally reported by me.

Once again, I got no feedback.

Shortly after this, Mr Jain covertly followed me after our regular Friday afternoon MDT meeting and confronted me outside the RLI operating theatres. I sent the following email about the encounter to Jodie Brownlie of Human Resources.

17th October 2014

Account of encounter with Mr A Jain, consultant urologist, 5.45pm 17th October.

> *I left the urology MDT meeting at about 5.30pm. I suspected and had been warned that Mr A J might try to waylay me and hence left with Mr J D, ostensibly to try and expedite an emergency case but in reality to make sure that I was not alone and without witnesses. I went with Mr J D to theatre, where we discussed the outstanding emergency case with the theatre co-ordinator. I left theatre on my own, leaving J D to prepare for his case and, to my dismay, realised that Mr A J had evidently followed and was waiting for me outside the theatre in an empty corridor, without witnesses. He approached me and said that we needed to sit down and discuss some of the issues with the urology Department face to face rather than submitting clinical incident forms and emails. He was intimidating and stood uncomfortably close so that I could smell his breath. I was not comfortable, but as I backed away, he closed the distance again. There was no direct physical threat, but I felt very uncomfortable. His voice was trembling and I could tell that he was very emotional. I replied that I had been asking for face-to-face discussions regarding relative departmental workloads and attitudes to emergency cases for over four years and had simply been mocked or scorned for suggesting that there were problems and gross imbalances. I said that things had got much worse since then and that some terrible things had happened within the department. To my surprise he acknowledged this point. I said that I felt that it was far too late now to finally start on informal chats and that I had a professional duty to share my very great concerns about clinical standards in the department. AJ replied that he also did ward rounds and found problems and irregularities too and could make*

statements and allegations about problems. I asked him to elaborate on this and to inform me of any clinical issues that he had found in relation to my own consultant work. He declined to answer this.

Mr AJ then talked about his previous Monday evening on-call that will be the subject of a forthcoming clinical incident. He claimed to have been very busy and said that the operating theatres had been constantly busy with high-priority clinical cases that took priority over the outstanding urology case that he had been tasked with carrying out (a frail patient with an obstructed kidney and candidal septicaemia). He said that because he was so busy trying to get his case to theatre, he had been unable to attend FGH to see the patient who had presented with an acute priapism.

I pointed out to him that the last elective case had finished at 6.40pm. The next emergency case had started at 8pm (a bleeding TURP, taken back to theatre by JD). This case finished at 9.30pm and was followed by an orthopaedic MUA (manipulation under anaesthesia) from 10pm – 11pm. There was plenty of space to have done his emergency case. I also pointed out that AJ had been contacted at 9.30pm to ask him if he would like to proceed with his case of an infected obstructed kidney ahead of the orthopaedic team. He had replied that it should be left for tomorrow's on-call consultant.

He accused me of checking up on him. I agreed that I had checked on ORMIS to see if his story was correct, and with the theatre co-ordinator. I told him that there was ample time for him to have done the outstanding emergency. I told him that I didn't trust his clinical judgement and that he exhibited abysmal levels of responsibility and ownership of acutely unwell patients. He replied that he worked hard and wasn't lazy 'like some people'. I asked him how that statement was compatible with the fact that historically I tended to follow his on-calls and several audits of emergency activity suggested that I had to shoulder about 400 – 600% of the out of hours workload that he took on.

He replied that the theatre team didn't allow him to do his share of emergency theatre work. He also stated that the priapism case at FGH has refused to come to RLI and that he couldn't be in two places at once. I suggested that the notes had recorded that it was AJ's decision to instruct the general surgical team to send the pa-

tient home rather than organising an immediate 'blue-light' transfer to RLI for a consultant delivered cavernosal washout and phenylephrine instillation, as should have been done. I suggested that instructing him to go home and to return at 7am for a taxi to RLI was completely inappropriate for a medical/surgical emergency. He blamed the general surgical team and said that he would be 'having words with them.' At this point he was standing very, very close to me and stated that he worked very hard and virtually never left any work for others to do. It occurred to me that he might be trying to provoke me into a rash statement and I recalled that he had spent much of the MDT (multi-disciplinary team meeting) fiddling with his iPhone under the desk. I strongly suspected at this point that he might be recording me. I felt it most appropriate to leave. I said something along the lines of ... 'Oh come off it Ash....' and then 'Sorry Ash, but I'm out of here.' I walked/ran downstairs. He made to follow but gave up after a few paces. I went home and prepared this report, handwriting it immediately and then formally typing it out on the 20th.

Peter Duffy.

The atmosphere in the department was truly awful at this point and on 17 November 2014 I emailed the Medical Director, Associate Medical Director and Clinical Director saying,

I had a brief but useful meeting with George today. I am worried sick about the state of the urology Dep't, esp' following the resignations of both Carl Rowbotham and Steve Douglas last week. I strongly fear that there are more to come and, as I said to George, 'I feel that the standards in the Dep't have deteriorated to the degree where if we were a Trust we'd be put in special measures.'

My fears were well founded and at around this time the Trust received an anonymous letter or email passed on by the Police, accusing me of bullying, racism and harming patients and stating that all BME (ethnic minority) doctors in the department were in fear of me.

I was never officially informed of this allegation. Far worse, I finally got to learn in March 2018 (just weeks before the April Tribunal and over three years after the event), the details of a meeting which also took place at the Royal Lancaster Infirmary in early December 2014 at the same time as the anonymous email/letter. At this covert meeting, identical allegations to those made to the Police were again asserted about me by Messrs Madhra, Jain and Naseem in the presence of the clinical lead, a senior manager and an external legal or employment adviser from the British Association of Physicians of Indian Origin (BAPIO) who had turned up unexpectedly. The minutes themselves were relatively anodyne but clearly transmitted the anger and frustration being directed at me behind my back in clear retaliation for my repeated and genuine concerns.

From the perspective of five years later, it is evident that as early as 2014, serious and in my opinion, defamatory retaliatory allegations were being made about me by the clinicians that I had expressed legitimate concerns about. These allegations including clear implications of racism by myself with correspondence at this point involving a Senior Employment Adviser from the Medical Defence Shield of the British Association of Physicians of Indian Origin (BAPIO), where I was again named without being aware of what was going on behind my back.

As I testified to the Tribunal in 2018, it is difficult to overstate the sheer toxicity of such allegations. I had been warned in my first few years in UHMB (after Mr Madhra's original allegations of prejudice when I first started raising concerns) that I must at all costs avoid an allegation of racism against me. I was told that such allegations, even if entirely unwarranted can destroy careers and that the NHS tends to regard the subject of a racism allegation as guilty by default.

Of course, I was completely unable to defend myself during this particular period, being entirely unaware that I was under attack or that such toxic three-way allegations were being made both internally and also to a powerful external and nationwide organisation which, for obvious reasons, is extremely sensitive to racism allegations.

Even the very existence of this meeting was with-held from me until some three months after my resignation in 2016 and I was denied any opportunity to review the actual physical record and minutes of the meeting right up until just weeks before the Employment Tribunal in 2018. The emails by which the reports on the meeting were circulated around and outside the Critical Care Division have never been divulged, despite the requirement that all evidence be declared prior to any litigation process. I doubt if I will ever find out the true extent to which these false allegations were spread around.

CHAPTER TEN

Avoidable death

BY THE BEGINNING OF 2015 we had what was to me a clearly avoidable death; something that I had both long dreaded and long predicted.

Mr A died in January 2015 from a stroke, sepsis (major infection) and in my opinion neglect, from what was a clear case of a blocked and infected ureteric stent (an artificial tube used to drain urine from the kidney to bladder) that was already overdue for a change and a blocked and infected kidney that we had been far too slow to drain.

The Royal College of Surgeons handbook on Surgical Standards stipulates that *Patients with septic shock and evidence of obstructive uropathy require immediate intervention within three hours of the decision to operate as delay increases mortality significantly.*

The sepsis was clearly evident by the Sunday lunchtime and all it required was a fifteen to twenty minute operation to give this dedicated husband and father a fighting chance of survival. With an operating theatre just yards away and with a consultant microbiologist advising surgery as soon as possible, it nevertheless took 48 hours to get this shocked, septic and desperately unwell patient to theatre. Even then, the person who performed the emergency surgery (myself) wasn't the person on-call or responsible for Mr A's care.

I first met Mr A and his family when he was a patient on the acute surgical unit. Some four days after this, I still recall my utter disbelief when, attending the surgical wards prior to carrying out a routine all-day operating list, I discovered that the chatty and friendly patient that I had spoken to some four days earlier was now critically ill in intensive care on a ventilator and inotropes (adrenaline-like drugs used intravenously to support a patient's blood pressure when they are shocked and/or septic). However, there was still no plan to actually tackle the source of the sepsis, get this patient to the operating theatre and drain the patient's blocked and infected kidney despite the fact that we were now well over 40 hours on from his diagnosis of severe sepsis. I had a distinct out-of-body moment, looking down on myself standing next to a nurse and the nurses' station in utter disbelief at what was happening, with the realisation dawning on me that it was probably already too late.

Tasked with preparing the four patients for the morning list as well as attending our pre-op checklist meeting, I vividly recall flying up and down the stairs at the back of the RLI Centenary Building, trying to co-ordinate and sweet-talk the emergency anaesthetist, X ray and radiographer, theatre and ICU so that we could attempt to get this desperately sick patient to theatre as an emergency over everyone's lunch-break. *If I break an ankle then I'll be no good to anyone*, was one of my more random thoughts as I vaulted down the steel tipped stairs, three to four at a time.

I'd hoped to get the patient down to X ray for a CT scan to check on whether the stent was heavily calcified (which might have made it difficult to change) and also to check the state of the other kidney but was told by the ICU consultant that the patient was far too unstable by this point to risk moving him anywhere other than the operating theatre for '…the fastest emergency stent change you've done in your life…'

The theatre and ICU teams excelled themselves and we did indeed get the patient to theatre as an emergency over lunch, with several members of the team volunteering to work for free through their allocated breaks. At the end of the operation I noted infected-looking urine to be draining from the fresh stent, confirming that the previous stent had indeed been blocked, with infected urine backing up in the kidney and also confirming the stent and kidney as being the source of the infection. By the end of the day the patient seemed cautiously better, although still critically ill.

Over the following 48 hours or so his renal (kidney) function normalised and his septic markers (blood tests) showed a dramatic improvement. I was beginning to hope that we hadn't left things too late when catastrophe struck. The patient developed dilated pupils, a subsequent CT scan showing a major stroke. To my despair and distress, he passed away shortly after the New Year of 2015.

Whilst I spoke out verbally at the time about the death, I was utterly despairing of standards in the urology department at this point and felt very alone and unsupported. I was well aware of my obligations to the patients and to the General Medical Council, but I'd had no feedback or support whatsoever from the previous incidents that I had submitted and by this point felt thoroughly hated and despised as a consequence of my repeated previous concerns and incident reports. Carl Rowbotham, consultant and Steve Douglas, urology nurse specialist had, as a consequence of standards in the department, handed in their resignations and there was clearly no desire amongst a small number of colleagues to improve our failings. Senior management appeared to me to be utterly complacent and apathetic. *Cover-up and carry-on* seemed to me to be the philosophy. I myself was simply too intimidated and frightened by the potential for more hostility and retaliation to put in a formal report regarding what was clearly an avoidable death and major incident following on from years of risk taking. To my intense shame, I allowed the incident to go past without formally alerting management, the GMC or the CQC about it.

Soon afterwards in perhaps late January or February of 2015 a nervous middle manager approached me 'strictly off the record' and, after much glancing over shoulders, informed me in a low monotone of rumours that the Police had received an anonymous allegation of racism and bullying against me. I was warned that my speaking up about clinical standards had made enemies; that I was being briefed against by several individuals and to *keep your head down and watch your back*. I was still completely unaware of the official meeting in December 2014 involving my colleagues, BAPIO and senior management and at which I had been labelled as a racist. I remained in ignorance of this until well after my resignation, never getting to see the official minutes until they had to be forced out of the Trust over three years later and only then after a preliminary Employment Tribunal hearing and legal order from the Judge.

We had a departmental meeting at about this time at the RLI where I insisted on presenting the very latest emergency turnover figures for the urology consultants (independently audited, incorporating the original figures for 2011-12 but now updated by the theatre manager and incorporating three years of data). In my opinion it screamed out that some individuals were shirking the emergency workload and passing it on to others. As soon as my turn came for the presentation, Mr Jain and Mr Naseem very deliberately stood up, turned their backs on me, put their coats on and walked out of the meeting. Eyebrows lifted and eyes swivelled as the rest of the department watched them silently leave the room without explanation or apology, only the click of the door latch breaking the brittle silence. The figures did indeed suggest that there a very wide variation indeed in the different consultants' attention to their emergency workload.

2011-12
Duffy – 50 cases
Mr A – 22
Mr B – 17
Mr C – 14
Mr D – 13
Mr E – 7

2012-13
Duffy – 59
Mr A – 35
Mr B – 16
Mr C – 24
Mr D – 32
Mr E – 26

2013-14
Duffy – 43*
Mr A – 46
Mr B – 11
Mr C – 16

Mr D – 31
Mr E – 12

*representing 9 months on-call, prevented from performing on-call duties by Occupational Health end Oct – end Jan

As though this were not enough we had another incident in February 2015 when, after being called to help out by an old friend and fellow surgical consultant from a different speciality, I had to go into the hospital over a weekend off and sort out a patient that Mr Jain, who at the time was on-call, had refused to operate on. It was another case of a blocked stent with, on this occasion, the patient leaking urine into the back of her abdomen, requiring an emergency scan and subsequently a very challenging emergency operation later that day. I spent most of my weekend off sorting out this patient, missing William's (our youngest son) school rugby match in the process and I think it very highly likely that she would have died within 24-48 hours without emergency intervention. Once again, the error of judgement was formally reported and once again there was no feedback whatsoever.

Dear ...,

Thank you for asking for my comments on the case of T relating to the events of Saturday 7th Feb.

I was still in bed when I was called by Mr ... at about 9.30am (I had had a busy on-call the night before). He told me that Mrs ... was a close family friend and that he'd just had her husband on the 'phone in tears, saying that Mrs ... had been seen by the on-call consultant, Mr A Jain and had been told that there was nothing that could be done and that there was no point in just carrying on changing stents. She had been virtually anuric (no urine output) since the removal of her catheter the previous lunchtime and now had a very distended and tender abdomen.

I already knew Mrs ... as I had changed her stents the previous weekend. She was in her mid-50's with metastatic breast cancer which the oncology team were hoping to treat with chemotherapy.

I was due to attend our youngest son's rugby match that morning, but I told … that I would go in and see her. I also told him that my relationship with Mr Jain was not good as a result of other, similar issues and he apologised for putting me in a difficult position. I considered 'phoning Mr Jain but decided against this for several reasons.

I went in and saw Mrs …. She was vomiting profusely, looked very unwell and had a very tender abdomen with no bowel sounds. A bladder scan had suggested a virtually empty bladder and it seemed highly likely that she had leaked and was continuing to leak urine from a pre-existing renal or ureteric defect that had been noted on several imaging tests over the preceding fortnight.

At this time Mr Jain saw me sitting at the nurses' desk, writing up the notes and came over, asking me what I was doing. I replied that I'd had a call asking me to review Mrs … and relayed by a family friend. I told Mr J that I was planning re-catheterisation, emergency blood tests and a non-contrast CT scan. He mumbled something along the lines of 'well I suppose we need to know what is going on.' It was a perfectly polite exchange but it was clear that he was very unhappy with my presence.

I supervised the catheterisation, noting that it drained almost nothing, spoke to the on-call radiologist and provisionally booked theatre, explaining to Mrs … my suspicions about a retro-peritoneal urine leak. I asked Mrs … if she was happy for me to hand her ongoing care and any possible surgery back to Mr J. She was adamant that she wished me to remain involved and would like me rather than anyone else to do any subsequent surgery.

As I was leaving the ward the sister in charge told me that Mr J had stated that he would submit a clinical incident form as I had interfered with the patient.

The blood tests showed a dramatically rising creatinine and CRP (inflammatory marker) consistent with a retro-peritoneal leak of infected urine, and I was 'phoned back by the on-call radiologist, stating that the CT scan confirmed this.

I therefore took Mrs … back to theatre that afternoon, carrying out a very challenging change of JJ stents which probably took about two hours, as the guide wire persistently passed through the defect into the retro-peritoneum rather than into the renal pelvis. Eventually I secured a correctly positioned stent, washed Mrs ...'s bladder out and left her with a catheter. I stayed in the hospital until it was clear that she had a good urine output, phoned several times that evening, went back in to see her the following day and Monday, and telephoned Dr ..., consultant medical oncologist on Monday morning to check that Mrs ... would be receiving her chemotherapy promptly before her disease progressed further.

I believe that my actions at all times were motivated by a desire to do the best thing for the patient and I believe that the patient might well have lost her life had I not intervened. I have had the regrettable experience in the recent past of handing over a patient requiring urgent surgery to Mr J, only for the surgery to be immediately cancelled and the patient sent home. I did not want to allow any possibility of this happening again, hence my decision to attend to Mrs ... in person and to remain directly engaged with her clinical care until I was satisfied that I had done all I could to optimise her condition.

Peter

This email was followed by this email exchange.

-----Original Message-----
From: ... (UHMB) [mailto:
Sent: 09 February 2015 21:04
To: Duffy Peter (UHMB)
Subject: Many Thanks

Hi Peter

Thanks very much for your help this week-end. I am sorry it put you in a difficult position with your colleague. A is so much better following your intervention and we are all grateful for you expertise and reassurance.

Best wishes,
...

-----Original Message-----
From: Duffy Peter (UHMB)
Sent: 10 February 2015 09:07
To: … (UHMB)
Subject: RE: Many Thanks

No problem. She certainly seemed much better yesterday. Creatinine has dropped from 264 to 83 yesterday with excellent urine output.

Spoke to Dr … y'day and understand that she's having a PICC line inserted tomorrow with a view to systemic chemotherapy.

Hope it all goes well and happy to be able to help.

Peter

-----Original Message-----
From: Duffy Peter (UHMB)
Sent: 10 February 2015 09:13
To: … (UHMB)
Subject: FW: Many Thanks

fyi

-----Original Message-----
From: … (UHMB)
Sent: 10 February 2015 09:20
To: Duffy Peter (UHMB)
Subject: RE: Many Thanks

Thanks Peter,
Good result.
…

From: Duffy Peter (UHMB)
Sent: 10 February 2015 11:30
To: … (UHMB)
Subject: RE: Many Thanks

Yes, but it wouldn't be if I hadn't intervened and spent my Saturday sorting it out…. :(

It was at this point (early 2015) that it became apparent that I had to leave the RLI as a result of the ongoing rudeness, aggression and hostility which had by now built up to unbearable levels and which was having a serious effect on my physical and mental health and sleep patterns. I was so frightened of retaliation that I'd even taken the precaution of fitting extra fire alarms alongside our front and back doors, so fearful was I of some middle-of-the-night act of revenge.

My extreme unhappiness and desire to get away from such an abusive environment was no secret and I was approached by NHS Scotland via a contact who had previously worked in UHMB (one of the original group of consultants who had spoken out about standards in Morecambe Bay) about a possible post in Oban, opening discussions about a potential move there.

Despite the awful working environment at the Royal Lancaster Infirmary there were still some good moments. Even at the worst of times I have never lost the sense of satisfaction that comes from completing a difficult procedure. Carl Rowbotham and I had always worked together on the difficult nephrectomies and just before he finally left the Trust we had one last chance to deploy our skills, faced with a young female patient with a truly huge left sided kidney cancer occupying most of the left side of her abdominal cavity.

This was certainly up there with the most challenging dozen or so operations that I have done in my life. Dealing with such huge tumours is all about exposure and access and it is sometimes necessary to deliberately open the patient's chest as well as the full length of the abdomen to gain enough exposure and control to deal with the kidney and surrounding organs safely (there are few sights more intimidating to an abdominal surgeon than seeing the chest open, lung collapsed and heart, sheathed in its pericardial coverings clearly beating away just inches from your operating site!).

In this case, having exposed the kidney and its surrounding perirenal fat, it turned out that the kidney was thoroughly stuck to all the surrounding organs including the colon (bowel), as well as being densely adherent to the aorta (the main artery from the heart), with very poor access to the main renal (kidney) artery, which was hidden under a huge, main renal vein. Not only is the main renal vein very easy to tear, but you can't ligate or tie it off to get at the artery behind as, if you do, the whole kidney swells hugely and begins to bleed heavily as blood is being pumped in and can't get out again!

If this were not bad enough, one of the characteristics of kidney tumours is that they can induce large extra blood vessels around the kidney, called *collateral* vessels. These can occur anywhere and can be both thin walled (and hence also easy to tear) and intimidatingly large. This unfortunate lady had them in abundance. Furthermore, even normal kidneys take about 20% of the heart's overall output between them (malignant kidneys a lot more) and if you accidentally tear these veins the bleeding can be truly terrifying and quickly life threatening. In such a case it is vital to have an experienced and reliable team to assist.

Carl and I probably spent three to four hours unpicking all the adhesions and meticulously clipping and tying off all the collateral vessels, coaxing the kidney out whilst Alan, one of our regular and very gifted anaesthetists, dripped in blood products and balanced the anaesthetic agents at the top end of the table, keeping up with the ongoing bleeding and maintaining the patient's stability. Luckily, in addition to Alan and Carl, I had Jill assisting, one of the regular urology theatre sisters. Jill was invariably excellent and utterly dependable, having an uncanny, almost spooky knack of handing me the instrument that I needed before I'd even decided what I wanted next.

On occasions like this, time seems to stand still and although you are working hard and utterly concentrating on the tiny area of tissue that you are working on, it can be almost relaxing. There are no phone calls or interruptions and the theatre staff are totally dedicated to doing everything to help you stay entirely focussed and to minimise distractions. Long operations like this can seem to fly past and it is only when the procedure is almost complete and the patient being closed up that you realise how intense it has been and how tired you are. Thankfully, in this case our efforts were rewarded with the renal artery and then finally the main renal vein tied off and divided and the kidney and surrounding tissues being cleanly lifted free of the incision, accompanied by a small cheer from the other theatre staff and trainees who had come to watch, and a sigh of relief from Carl, myself, Jill and Alan.

I'd like to think that Carl, Jill, Alan and I made a good team, having carried out several dozens of such procedures during our time together. With Carl's leaving date now just days away, I was deeply upset that what had been such a highly performing team over the previous decade was now irreversibly breaking up.

It was around this point that a move back to Furness General Hospital in South Cumbria was mooted for me. At the time the Trust was employing long term agency locum consultants of variable quality to cover Mr Madhra's absence. Including agency costs, it was rumoured that such locums were costing between a quarter and half a million pounds a year. Colin, as clinical lead, had previously proposed trying to attract a senior full time regular NHS consultant instead, suggesting an annual gross salary of around £200,000 to include commuting time and expenses. This would save significant money whilst in return for such a financial commitment the department would be able to demand a very arduous working week in excess of sixty hours with a full commitment both to quality and quantity of service. The new appointee would also be expected to take full responsibility for heading up and driving forward the service in South West Cumbria.

As my commitment to follow Carl and Steve's resignations hardened and the news of my unhappiness spread, a number of individuals approached me to suggest that a swift move to Barrow might resolve many of my issues. In a meeting in March 2015 I agreed in principle to place my ongoing negotiations with NHS Highlands and Islands on ice whilst we tried to work out an alternative that might enable me to stay in the Trust. I emailed the Scottish Trust to say:

> *In essence, I will be based in Furness General Hospital (rather than Lancaster), offered travel time and expenses, taken off the on-call rota and given a substantial pay rise (they were talking £200K!).*

At this point, some 10 years after his appointment, Carl Rowbotham served out what remained of his resignation notice together with our long serving urology nurse specialist, Steve Douglas. Relationships had by now deteriorated, in what was left of the department, to the point where the Critical Care Division called in two clinical psychologists to try and tackle the 'dysfunctional behaviour'. At this point I was, of course, still unaware of the seriousness and extent of the racism allegations against myself.

We had several group meetings with the clinical psychologists, the last being in March 2015. We concluded by all formally agreeing and promising to treat each other and the patients with politeness and respect. The remaining individuals after Carl and Steve's resignations, formally agreed to try and work together as a team.

Mr Naseem went off on study leave immediately after the meeting broke up. On his very first morning back he delivered such an aggressive and offensive phone call that I rang up Colin and told him that I had to leave UHMB altogether or be transferred away from Lancaster immediately to get away from such behaviour. The call came through just as I was about to start my afternoon's outpatient clinic.

The latter part of the call was witnessed by my then secretary, one of our clinical nurse specialists and the clinic nurse for the afternoon.

Thankfully, the nurse was a regular colleague and well used to my way of working. Unsettled to the point of distraction by the phone call, I repeatedly and dangerously forgot to write in notes, fill in request forms and dictate letters that afternoon. Mercifully, my nursing colleague patiently jogged my memory and pointed out my repeated errors and we staggered through what seemed like a never ending clinic without any major omissions or mistakes.

Whilst Mr Naseem did ring back later to apologise, with the call coming just days after we'd all pledged to be polite and respectful to each other, the damage was well and truly done.

To Colin's great credit he managed to persuade me to not resign with immediate effect and arranged my almost immediate transfer to FGH. I started there at the beginning of April 2015 on what I understood to be an agreement of £200,000 a year in exchange for a working week which would be very intensive, would never go below 60 hours per week and would exceed this quite significantly on occasions. Provisionally, the arrangement was for me to be paid for 48 hours at regular rates and to supplement this by paying me weekly for an extra 10 hours at the 'AAS' (Additional activity session) rate of £500 a session.

It was clear from the start that we'd rather undershoot the £200,000 gross that had originally been proposed but a review after six months was agreed. I accepted the plan, and was moved over to FGH at about 48 hours' notice. The swift and decisive action undoubtedly saved my career within Morecambe Bay, although of course this proved to be little more than a stay of execution.

CHAPTER ELEVEN

Catch 22
Disobedience to HM Coroner

FOR MY FIRST FEW MONTHS I was very happy indeed at Furness General Hospital. I had escaped from an immensely hostile environment at the RLI and thoroughly enjoyed reforming old friendships with staff that I had worked with ten to fifteen years before, in my earlier years with Richard Wilson. Although there were a few very occasional encounters with Mr Naseem and Mr Jain, I felt very much more secure. For several months I was paid properly in line with what had been agreed and overall, I was happy to still have a job within the Trust that I had always had a vocation to work in. I was relieved to have left behind the clinically very dangerous and personally toxic environment of the RLI. My formal appraisal from 2014-15 noted:

> I feel much more comfortable in my current role. As hinted at above, I have endured difficult relationships with colleagues, with prompt, competent treatment of urological emergencies being a particular area of difficulty. In my new role, (without any formal on-call commitment) I feel much more comfortable and the potential for conflict is much reduced.

My appraiser noted:

> Mr Duffy recognises that there are issues within the department regarding this domain. In the past he has tried to resolve these without success at some cost to his health. Now that he has moved post

to FGH he has effectively removed himself from conflict which he has seen as the only solution.

It seemed at this point that I'd fallen on my feet. But in around May 2015 a seemingly innocent email arrived which nevertheless signalled the beginning of the end of my career and vocation within Morecambe Bay and the wider NHS.

The email was from the Trust's legal department and asked me to attend a Coroner's inquest into the death of patient A, the emergency case that I'd taken to theatre over lunch at the RLI after Christmas 2014.

I didn't need to be reminded of the facts. Mr A's death had continued to trouble a good number of us in the urology department for months afterwards and had been widely and repeatedly discussed as a clearly avoidable disaster. Now I was being asked to go and give evidence under oath to the Coroner about his death, a death which I and other colleagues still regarded as being clearly avoidable, the result of terrible neglect and yet, which equally and clearly hadn't triggered any changes in standards in the department. I'd already quietly noted that, despite the fact that **_all_** post-operative NHS surgical deaths are supposed to be discussed in regular surgical M&M meetings (Morbidity and Mortality meetings), Mr A's death had never been submitted for review or discussed by the consultants who had been in charge of his care at any of the meetings that had followed his death. A number of the department had quietly behind the backs of hands discussed a virtually identical case from Bradford where the consultant urological surgeon in question had been jailed for over a year for gross negligence manslaughter.

This felt like a medical version of the classic Catch 22 situation.

Being straightforward and honest with the Coroner would almost certainly trigger huge acrimony and retaliation against me, probably an investigation and possibly even involvement of a regulatory organisation like the GMC or CQC. However, if I was less than honest then I'd be misleading the Coroner and the grieving family whilst of course also being under oath. I was well aware of the duty placed upon doctors to be honest and forthright in their professional dealings and in particular the duty to speak up to protect patients' lives and well-being.

Finally, it was clear that the Coroner would focus in like a laser on the huge and easily avoidable 48 hour delay in changing Mr A's blocked and infected stent once he had become severely septic; an omission which, to any experienced urological surgeon, stood out like a sore thumb.

A compromise (and possible cowardly way out of the Catch 22) was if someone else was prepared to attend the Court in my place. I therefore emailed my two Lancaster colleagues who had been on-call during the Christmas weekend and following week to ask if they would attend instead.

Both declined to answer and I was therefore left with no alternative but to attend.

I had a clear choice. Under oath I could either prevaricate and bluster, giving bland, uninformative answers, lead the Coroner off in the wrong direction and generally give the overall impression that everyone had vaguely done their best and this was an unavoidable tragedy... Or I could tell the truth.

Drafting out my statement at the secretaries' workstation several days before the inquest, I became aware of one of my colleagues looming rather menacingly over the desk.

What are you planning on telling the Coroner?

The truth, was the reply.

Preparing a straightforward statement, I attended Lancaster Coroner's Court just a few days later, being questioned under oath by the Coroner.

The Coroner, as predicted, was clearly very concerned about the delayed stent change and asked me point-blank if I would have changed the stent as an emergency if I'd been on-call on the Sunday. With a heavy heart and intense sense of foreboding I told her "yes". She asked me if there was a departmental meeting where the case could be discussed and a departmental speciality consensus reached on whether the stent should indeed have been changed on that Sunday as an emergency. I replied that, as is required of each department in the NHS, we had a monthly Morbidity and Mortality (M&M) meeting, at that time being chaired and organised by Mr Naseem at which all of the deaths under our care were supposed to be discussed. Asked if the case had already been presented and what the conclusions had been (as above, it is required practice that all post-operative hospital deaths are discussed in the relevant M&M meeting), I told her that the case had never been listed for discussion.

The Coroner subsequently produced a 'narrative' verdict:

> [Patient A] *died on 2 January 2015 at Royal Lancaster Infirmary as a result of a stroke he suffered on 1 January 2015 which was contributed to by his underlying medical conditions and the development of urosepsis following missed opportunities to change his ureteric stent.*

She formally ordered that I should submit a clinical incident and that we as a department should discuss the case at our next M&M meeting. She instructed me to compile a second report of the departmental conclusions and consensus opinion from the M&M meeting and return this to her. After questioning me on dates she extended the deadline for me to submit a subsequent report to beyond the date of the next M&M meeting, specifically to allow this to happen.

At our next M&M meeting I took the notes along and prepared for the case to be discussed as per the Coroner's orders. As I described to the Tribunal, as soon as I walked into the M&M meeting room with Mr A's very recognisable notes under my arm (in true NHS fashion they were in a tatty old supermarket shopping bag and held together with elastic bands) my two colleagues, Mr Jain and Mr Naseem both immediately stated very bluntly 'We are not discussing that case.'

I pointed out that the Coroner had given us a direct order and a deadline but was again met with a repeated point-blank refusal to allow the case to be discussed. I carefully informed the group that we were about to knowingly disobey HM Coroner and that we could be held as being in contempt as this was a direct and unequivocal order, given in the Coroner's Court in session. However, after a further blunt refusal I clearly had no choice but to give in. Mr Naseem was the chair of the M&M meeting and I felt that I could do nothing more than accede to his instructions.

After the Morbidity and Mortality meeting was over, my two colleagues then insisted that instead of complying with the Coroner's orders, the three of us who had been involved in this case should prepare separate reports. These would then be combined into a single report to the Coroner, thereby outnumbering me 2:1 and of course, neatly excluding the opinions of all the other urological surgery experts in the department, something that HM Coroner had clearly been at pains to avoid.

I vigorously protested about this, stating in an email on 12th June:

> For the record, I very definitely did **not** agree with the decision not to discuss [Patient A] in the Morbidity and Mortality meeting as is suggested below.... I pointed out several times [to the M&M meeting] as forcefully as I could that the Coroner's Court is a Court of Law, that the Coroner's instructions are, I presume, legally binding and that we were knowingly ignoring these instructions. I even pointed out that (in theory at least) we could be in contempt of court by wilfully or knowingly declining to co-operate with the Coroner's clear instructions.
>
> I've phoned the Coroner's officer just to check that my recollection of the Coroner's instructions was accurate. She was in court herself that day....
>
> The Coroner's officer clearly recalls the instruction that the case be discussed at this next meeting and also recalls that the deadline for the report was extended to the end of June to allow a margin of time after the M&M meeting for the department's conclusions at the M&M meeting to be included in the final report.
>
> As we've completely failed to follow the Coroner's clear instructions and do not have another M&M meeting until after the Coroner's deadline has expired, I'd welcome ...'s advice on where we go from here.

I tried to warn the Coroner via the Coroner's officer that a cover-up was going on but in the meantime Morecambe Bay's legal office intervened and the Coroner's office seemed to prefer to deal with the issue through them. An email to the Coroner (produced by Morecambe Bay in evidence to the Tribunal and not previously seen by myself), gave the impression that I and the Trust were together pushing for an early resolution to the case via a Root Cause Analysis (RCA) meeting. In fact I was vehemently opposed to this as it meant continuing to disobey both the order given to me by HM Coroner and NHS protocol.

Both Mr Duffy and the Trust are anxious to action the Area Coroner's request and we would be grateful if you could confirm with [the Coroner] *that this approach would be acceptable to her.*

The Coroner acceded to the suggestions of Morecambe Bay's legal office, presumably without being aware that I had voiced my complete and utter opposition to the above plan and had also voiced my concern that there appeared to be a determination not to discuss the case with the rest of the urology department and to continue to hide the case from formal review in the M&M meeting.

At this juncture, it is important to point out that the only group of clinicians in Morecambe Bay knowledgeable enough to meaningfully comment on this very specialist area of urological emergency case management was in the urology department. In a similar vein, I was concerned that this move away from the Coroner's clear and logical instructions would leave me isolated, without the support of the other members of the department and with only my opinion against that of two of my colleagues.

A colleague also expressed his concerns over the process, stating:

I also think that a divisionally led RCA (Root Cause Analysis) may not be appropriate for such complex specialist case.... I would suggest obtaining an independent expert urology specialist opinion based on the notes and the reports from my three consultant colleagues.

My reply noted:

I also feel that an outside expert opinion would be warranted. The case chiefly revolves around the emergency surgical care of a sick and deteriorating man with obstructive urosepsis. Any non-urology clinician expected to comment on the case should at least have some recent hands-on experience of such quite uncommon cases, otherwise we'll compromise the whole process.

Despite these well-justified concerns, the division's determination to avoid departmental discussion and to keep the investigation *in-house*, away from any other urological surgeons and under wraps ultimately prevailed, with subsequent events completely convincing me that there was a thorough on-going cover-up underway.

Mr Jain, Mr Naseem and I were instructed to prepare and share our three reports with each other prior to the RCA meeting and were categorically and repeatedly promised that we would all get the opportunity to scrutinise and request amendments to the subsequent RCA report before it was passed to the Coroner. Also, that it would not be passed on until we were all satisfied that it was an accurate and faithful representation of the truth.

In the event, not a single one of these assurances was honoured. I never got to see Mr Jain's report before it was submitted, nor was I ever even aware that Mr Naseem had submitted a second report on the avoidable death until I discovered it to my astonishment in the Tribunal bundle of evidence in early March 2018, nearly two years later!

The minutes of the highly secretive RCA meeting itself were never disclosed, even to the 2018 Tribunal, and the RCA meeting itself seemed to me to be a complete travesty as the departmental lead (Mr Cutting) was excluded and replaced by a non-urological surgeon as chair who was a friend of both Mr Jain and Mr Naseem. Although the chair and associate chair of the RCA meeting had some knowledge of urology and sepsis respectively, they both privately confided in me that they had no idea whatsoever about how to manage this highly specialist area of closed organ urinary sepsis. Therefore, as I'd feared and predicted, there was no departmental representation or specialist urological opinion available for what was a complex and important surgical investigation into an avoidable death through neglect. Furthermore, despite repeated promises that this wouldn't happen, the resulting and, in my opinion, hopelessly inadequate RCA report was then submitted directly to the Coroner without my being able to see it or give an opinion on its conclusions.

In the meantime, the briefings against me resumed, with documents submitted to the April 2018 Tribunal hearing showing further evidence of Mr Jain covertly accusing me of racism against the Asian consultants (from an email on 22 July 2015 that I was completely unaware of). I can't quantify how much verbal briefing there was against me at this time but I was told afterwards that it was significant. Also, at about the same time Belinda, my loyal and long-standing urology line manager was moved to orthopaedics and was replaced by a new manager called Louise, although Belinda remained in the background, providing support for some months after.

The completed RCA report on Mr A's death was submitted directly to the Coroner on 30ᵗʰ July 2015 without, as was promised, any attempt to share it with me or allow me to validate its conclusions.

I was by now in no doubt whatsoever as to what was going on.

Noting that the RCA completely failed to address the 48 hour delay in emergency surgery, I displayed my dismay at the submission of the report on the 31ˢᵗ July, saying:

Dear …,

Thank you for copying me into this. I very much regret that it has been forwarded to the coroner without prior circulation to the relevant individuals. I emphatically reject the contents, believing that the report is unbalanced, out of context, full of trivialities and distractions and ignores the Coroner's requests and substantive urological service failings that probably contributed to Mr A's sad demise.

I'd provided a comprehensive report to the RCA meeting, which was backed up with facts and which quoted from several learned texts and expert individuals on the subject of the emergency management of obstructive urosepsis.

The European Association of Urology states that:

> *Severe sepsis is a severe situation with a reported mortality rate of 20-42% and goes on to stipulate that ....drainage of any obstruction in the urinary tract and removal of foreign bodies, should lead to resolution of symptoms and recovery. This condition is an absolute emergency.*

Similarly, I quoted an excellent review article from the Memorial University of Newfoundland, *What to do about Obstructive Urosepsis:*

> *With obstructive urosepsis, the immediate goal is to stabilize the patient and intervene as soon as possible to ensure drainage of the obstructed, infected system.*

Campbell's Urology, the definitive 4,000 page urological surgery text, states that:

> *The prompt relief of obstruction is emergently required in cases of uraemia or sepsis.*

The definition of emergently is 'an additional expletive for emergency'! This patient had both sepsis and uraemia.

No evidence to justify the 48 hour delay or to support non-surgical 'medical' management of these kinds of emergencies was offered by my colleagues.

Despite this, the subsequent RCA report made no attempt whatsoever to address the two day wait for emergency surgery and appeared to completely ignore the powerful impartial expert evidence that I had provided.

I was so convinced at this point that a concerted cover-up was going on that for the first time I spoke to the General Medical Council's help-line for advice. They were extremely concerned and assured me that they'd be looking into my concerns over the situation with considerable urgency. However, they stipulated that they could only investigate named doctors and specific incidents, errors and deaths.

Having told the GMC all about my concerns and particularly about the case of Patient A, the failure to discuss the case in the M&M meeting, the issues over the RCA report and my misgivings over a divisional cover-up, I could barely think of anything else for the next 24 hours. Driven to distraction by worry and after a night spent agonising over the possible consequences and backlash over my candour, I was so anxious over what I had done that I emailed back the following day:

31st July 2015

Dear Sir or Madam,

I spoke to a very helpful lady yesterday about my concerns regarding personal and professional standards relating to some of my consultant urology colleagues at the University Hospitals of Morecambe Bay NHS Trust.

Since the conversation I have agonised over my decision to phone you. Although I was entirely honest during the call and continue to believe that the department is deeply dysfunctional and unsafe; in the end I have decided that the personal cost to myself of reporting these individuals is likely to be too high, particularly as the incidents that I detailed are ones that I was intimately involved in and it will be very easy for the erring consultants to figure out who reported them and to exact their revenge again.

I'd be grateful if I could therefore withdraw my concerns unequivocally, and I apologise for wasting your time.

Yours faithfully,
Peter Duffy.
3302114

However, I continued my protests from within Morecambe Bay and sent the following email on 3rd August 2015:

Dear ... and ...,

I've taken the weekend to consider the RCA report into the demise of Mr A and I'd be grateful if I could have an urgent conversation with you. I could not be more concerned about both the content of the report and the impact that this will have on the Coroner's ultimate conclusions.

By far and away the greatest failing in our management of the Mr A case was the failure, once sepsis was clearly demonstrated, to treat the case as an immediate surgical emergency. Nowhere does the report tackle or even acknowledge this wholly unacceptable delay in definitive management; indeed I cannot see one single point in the RCA report that reflects the concerns that I expressed in my own second report. It is as if my own opinions on the case do not exist.

Even more importantly, this is not an isolated case. Quite incredibly, even since the pretty gross mismanagement of the Mr A case came to light, we have had more cases of conservative management of obstructive urosepsis, with immediate, potentially lifesaving surgical intervention failing to be instituted and the patient being left for someone else to sort out. On two occasions in recent weeks I have had to step in (despite not being on-call or doing emergency work in my current role) and ensure that emergency surgery was promptly carried out, on one occasion staying at FGH until after 2am to ensure that the patient was given the required surgery.

We have lost at least one other patient in recent years on top of the Mr A case from inadequately treated urosepsis and more lives may well be lost in the future unless some individuals in the department start to take the issue of obstructive urosepsis and the wider ownership and prioritisation of urological emergencies more seriously. To my very intense anger and frustration, I have brought up the issue of delayed emergency treatment of our sicker inpatients time after time, and have pointed out over and over again all the way back to around 2010 the huge variation in emergency operative intervention rates among different consultants.

Please can I suggest that the RCA report is unconditionally and immediately withdrawn? If it is not, then I believe that we may be accused of fundamentally misleading the Coroner and family as to a major contributory cause of Mr A's death. We cannot afford to have this happen, especially after the Trust was found to have distorted evidence to the coroner in the Joshua Titcombe case [which led to the Morecambe Bay midwifery scandal]. *There are, of course, a number of other worrisome parallels with the JT case and I feel very strongly that the Trust needs to act swiftly and decisively before the situation escalates further.*

Please find attached my 2nd report to the RCA committee.

Yours sincerely,

The urgent conversation, of course, never took place and by this point my anxiety was worsened further by the knowledge that the report into the Morecambe Bay Investigation regarding the well-publicised midwifery scandal had been published just a few months earlier in May 2015. This was a top level investigation into dangerous and sometimes lethal practice in the midwifery department at Furness General Hospital, where national standards of care had been ignored and where a culture of cover-up and complacency had developed. The investigation had been carried out by the highly respected Dr Bill Kirkup, revealing that several members of staff had been heavily promoting natural childbirth at pretty much any cost. The service was described as being *beset by a culture of denial, collusion and incompetence,* with work inside the unit found to be *seriously dysfunctional,* with *poor levels of clinical competence, extremely poor working relationships, and a determination among certain midwives to pursue normal childbirth regardless of the consequences.*

Several of the midwives at FGH were so cavalier they became known as 'the musketeers'.

Dr Kirkup found that front-line staff were responsible for *inappropriate and unsafe care* and that the response to potentially fatal incidents by the trust hierarchy was *grossly deficient, with repeated failure to investigate properly and learn lessons.* He went on to point out that this *lethal mix of factors had led to twenty instances of significant or major failures of care at FGH, associated with three maternal deaths and the deaths of sixteen babies at or shortly after birth.*

An investigation into the death was described as being both *rudimentary* and *over protective of staff* and *failed to identify and deal with the underlying problems.*

The report went on to detail that between 2006 and 2008 there was a series of further *missed opportunities*.

All showed evidence of the same problems of *poor clinical competence, insufficient recognition of risk, inappropriate pursuit of natural childbirth and failures of team-working.*

To make matters worse, Dr Kirkup's investigators found evidence of *inappropriate distortion* in the preparation for a Coroner's inquest, with the circulation of *what we could only describe as model answers* in what appeared to be a conscious attempt to deflect the Coroner's investigations into the case.

Of course, these were all common factors within the urological surgery department as well. We too had also a very long history of dangerous behaviour within the department with neglect of emergency cases being of particular concern. The emergency theatre turnover figures for our speciality clearly showed a massive disparity between the intervention rates of different consultants going back years, with the treatment of urological sepsis and infections seeming to be particularly poor and not in keeping with national and international minimum standards. We also had at least one previous death from very poorly managed sepsis back in about 2011 and a good many incidents that could easily have ended in avoidable deaths, had I and others not stepped in to take charge. There were other incidents of severe and avoidable harm to patients and numerous warnings that had been ignored. Finally, here we were, just months after Dr Kirkup's savagely and justifiably critical report, not so much preparing model answers for the Coroner's Court, but (considerably worse), refusing point-blank to comply with a direct order from HM Coroner. All this despite the criticism made of the Trust over just such a sequence of events in the midwifery department only a few months earlier.

It was clear that we were making exactly the same mistakes again.

A colleague commented on the RCA report in a similar vein:

> *I think that the conclusion(s) misses the main key failing that this patient had an infected obstructed kidney. The infection and*

sepsis were not going to improve as long as the infected, blocked stent was still in situ.

The fact is that if this man had been taken to theatre earlier, he may not have gone on to die. This is a tragedy and as a Trust we should be committed to trying to ensure that such an event never happens again.

I would suggest that the Coroner is contacted and that we as a Trust promise to get an urgent external expert urologist review of the case which is then reported back to her and the patient's family.

Of course, none of this happened and I agonised and endured near sleepless nights and distracted days for nearly a month.

What was I to do now? My professional duty to the patients, relatives and my profession was brutally clear, but if I discharged such duties then it was equally clear that I'd be jeopardising the good names and reputations of not only the Trust itself but the whole executive board which was, of course, still busy congratulating itself about recently escaping from 'Special Measures', imposed after the scandal, errors and cover-ups of the midwifery era and assuring all and sundry that such errors and cover-ups couldn't happen again.

I observed in an email to a colleague:

I'm in no doubt that there's a determined attempt going on to deceive the Coroner and family and cover-up some pretty gross failings.

Another email sent by a colleague in the urology department at the time read:

Having reviewed the case carefully, I think that it was medically negligent that this patient was not taken to theatre earlier than they were and that the delay may well have led to the patient dying prematurely.

Acutely aware of the penalty that my family and I might end up paying for my decision to tell the Coroner the truth and discharge my duty of care and candour and, having widely discussing the issues with a good number of colleagues from both the department and the wider Trust, I called the Care Quality Commission on 25th August. I reported both my own and their concerns and the fact that we seemed to be repeating the very same sequence of clinical and managerial errors that had characterised the midwifery department at FGH. In particular, I emphasised my worries that we had had a string of very similar errors in the department culminating in an avoidable death from neglect, a cover-up and in my opinion, an attempt to mislead, misinform and disobey the Coroner.

This was all documented in the CQC's timeline from 2015-16 where I was described as being *terrified* that it might end my career in the NHS.

This was certainly true.

I remember my voice shaking so much that I could barely make myself understood by the CQC employee on the other end of the phone. I made the call from my mobile phone in my car, parked in the FGH car park as I was so scared of being overheard. It was lunchtime and the dark blue Fiesta had been standing in the sun all morning. Blazing hot and with the sweat tricking down my neck and chest, I nevertheless locked myself into the baking vehicle, making sure all the windows were firmly closed before daring to make the call. I was well aware of the appallingly high price paid by other NHS whistle-blowers and their families and the kind of plausibly deniable career 'accidents' that had befallen so many others who had come before me in the National Health Service. Despite the suffocating heat, I needed the psychological safety of being locked in the oven-like car before I dared place the call.

I'd approached a good number of friends and colleagues about whether I should report my concerns to the CQC. Whilst being entirely supportive, not one single one failed to warn me in graphic language of the potential career consequences. Once again, it appeared that Morecambe Bay had tolerated a string of errors, with patients' lives being risked, direct harm to patients, episodes of neglect and an overwhelming culture of lassitude, cover-up, deceit, bullying and complacency. *Cover-up and carry-on* was back as the organisational norm. Now it was my job and professional obligation to pass this information outside the organisation.

Vengeance would not be short, in either time or measure.

CHAPTER TWELVE

The Care Quality Commission

THE CQC WERE NOT to be rushed and I had a number of subsequent conversations with them over the summer of 2015. Urging them to speak to a broad cross-section of the department, I even provided a detailed list of colleagues including mobile phone numbers so that my concerns could be corroborated and independently verified. Unfortunately and to my extreme frustration, not a single member of the department was spoken to. Neither was anyone else from the department prepared to contact the CQC, all my contacts and confidantes being acutely aware of the retaliation that might befall them.

Increasingly, I was on my own.

The CQC finally discussed my concerns with UHMB's senior management in October 2015. I was warned of the forthcoming investigation and was well aware that the CQC had not sought independent corroboration from within the department. I was worried sick and again had a return of my ventricular ectopics. I was convinced that UHMB and in particular the Critical Care Division would, as a consequence of my previous emails, immediately figure out who had reported the issues and that with the reputation of the executive and particularly the Critical Care Division at stake, I would be targeted for swift revenge and retaliation.

After nearly 30 years of regular earnings, opening my end-of-the-month payslip was about as humdrum and routine as getting out of bed in the morning. However, at the end of October 2015 I tore open the slip with an overwhelming sense of apprehension. Having been punished once before by the Critical Care Division with an unauthorised pay cut after speaking out about NHS standards, I had a dread sense of *deja-vu*. Sure enough, 40+ hours of overtime pay had vanished from my earnings. The division without any explanation, had abruptly halted my ten hours a week of overtime pay, amounting to a pay cut of £1,000 per week whilst continuing to pay AAS sessional monies to all the other consultants.

It was in my opinion very effective retaliation. Morecambe Bay couldn't threaten me directly as I was just doing my job. They couldn't immediately cut my regular pay without my permission or demote me, nor could they immediately and legally alter my terms and conditions unilaterally (although they threatened to do so later). However, a refusal to pay me for the overtime work left me helpless, with any link to my discussions with the CQC being easily deniable (as I was to learn later in the Employment Tribunal).

As all this was going on I had my first meeting with Dr David Walker, the new Medical Director, informing him of my great fears about the department and the previous events detailed above. He agreed with my concerns, stating that getting the department sorted out was one of his top priorities. I also expressed my concerns that meetings had been going on between him, Mr Jain, Mr Madhra and Mr Naseem. I was worried that they might have been briefing against me or might even have made retaliatory allegations against me but was comprehensively reassured that, although such meetings had gone on, they were purely about Trust matters and nothing to do with me or with the department.

Despite all the ongoing issues over clinical standards and the fact that there was an ongoing interest in clinical safety within the department from the Coroner, at around this time and to my utter disbelief, there were two more critical clinical errors and, in my opinion, cover-ups.

Two patients, each with a single kidney, underwent what, in my and the rest of the department's opinion were inadequately completed procedures. The surgeon failed to protect the single kidneys by inserting a ureteric stent at the end of the procedure as is considered routine practice in urological surgery.

The cases in question were ureteroscopies as described earlier. This procedure involves inserting a very fine scope up the ureter towards and sometimes as far as the kidney. The scope is tiny, perhaps the size of a small but very long drinking straw, but so are the ureters themselves. It is almost inevitable that there will be a degree of trauma and swelling post-operatively, known as 'oedema' in medical terms.

Of course, in patients with two normal kidneys this isn't so critical, as even if one ureter swells and blocks the kidney temporarily after ureteroscopy, the patient can rely on the other kidney. However, if the patient has only one kidney (or the procedure is done on both kidneys or ureters) then the swelling can be life-threatening as the ureters can block and obstruct the drainage of urine, precipitating renal (kidney) failure. The absolute rule under these circumstances (ureteroscoping a single kidney or both kidneys at the same time) is to pass a ureteric stent (a small internal silicone tube that sits inside the ureter) at the end of the procedure to protect the kidney(s) from blockage and failure.

Both these patients had ureteroscopies on single kidneys on the same operating list and had no stent passed at the end of the procedure. Both patients were then discharged home. Both were subsequently readmitted as emergencies with both patients predictably going into renal (kidney) failure and requiring further emergency operations to complete their procedures. I carried out one emergency procedure, the other being performed by a very capable locum surgeon at the time before the patient was transferred to my care. Either or both patients could have died. This was yet another incident that was reported to my contact in the CQC.

The department discussed their cases in the next M&M meeting in October 2015. The surgeon in question, Mr Jain, was adamant that both patients had met pre-operatively and agreed together to refuse to have the stents inserted despite being repeatedly warned of the potential consequences. This seemed highly unlikely (they didn't know each other and were male and female. The day-surgery ward rigorously separates the patients according to gender and NHS regulations). A significant number of the attendees expressed extreme scepticism after the meeting broke up and were concerned that those attending M&M meeting had been fundamentally misled.

As I had looked after and been responsible for both patients and had performed the emergency surgery on one of them, it was agreed that I ought to contact them both to determine whether or not Mr Jain's version of events was correct and report this to the division if his version proved to be misleading.

Having spoken to the two patients over the phone one evening a few days later, I established that neither patient had refused stents or had any knowledge of the other. I reported this on to the division.

Shortly after this I took a call from the Clinical Director, Ms Joshi:

I'm going to ask you a question. I'm only going to ask it once and I want you to think long and hard before you answer it.

She was clearly very angry and I vividly recall the opening statement as though it were yesterday. She then went on to ask if I had contacted the two patients in question by telephone. She seemed confident that I would deny it and appeared rather wrong footed when I immediately told her that I didn't need to think about it and yes, of course I had. Despite defending myself and my actions on the basis that I was acting on clinical concerns and on behalf of the wider department, it was clear that my actions were deeply disapproved of and that I had caused serious problems for the Critical Care Division. Once again, there was no feedback.

Between October and November 2015 a lot of things happened and it is difficult to sort them out into their exact chronological order. Firstly on October 2nd we all received a group PDF email and formal written letter from Ms Joshi stating amongst other things:

I trust you are all in agreement with the importance of timely and urgent management of an obstructed infected kidney which is a urological emergency. The word 'emergency' means a serious, un-expected, and often dangerous situation requiring immediate action or management. The de-obstruction of an obstructed infected kidney MUST be performed as soon as safely possible for a patient. This also includes blocked/infected stents in situ. If there are genuine clinical reasons why de-obstruction via stenting (nephrostomy) is not undertaken as an emergency then this has to be clearly documented in the clinical notes.

In future any urologist found to be failing in their duty of care in this regard will face an investigation with the Medical Director which may proceed to disciplinary action and reporting to the GMC.

Yours sincerely,
Ameeta Joshi, Clinical Director Surgery & Critical Care.

This was clearly as a consequence of the avoidable death of Patient A that I had expressed concerns about to the CQC.

Despite this, the errors continued. On 5th October I wrote to the Clinical Director:

It is noteworthy that (unbelievably) we had yet another incident, just a few weeks ago where a case of obstructive urosepsis was reported to the on-call consultant who again advised antibiotics, IV fluids and observation overnight, possibly theatre the following day, but no firm plan for definitive surgical intervention. Luckily the case happened at FGH, I rang up at the end of the day to check about any new admissions, found out the circumstances and, with …'s help was able to institute emergency surgical intervention (… went over and stented that evening). I understand that yet another CI was submitted.

This was another immediate emergency which should have been dealt with within the Royal College three hour standard. Yet again there was no feedback.

This was followed by even more errors later that year where I wrote:

Had a pre-NY drink with my ex colleagues last night. Yet another case of an inadequately managed infected obstructed kidney has just occurred, taking 5 days to get to surgery (Royal College standard is 3 hours). No one is prepared to take it further as they're all terrified of speaking out now after what has happened to me….

I continued…, *I'm at a loss to know where we go from here, as we're still treating these patients as semi-elective cases, and we're clearly going to get another avoidable death, probably sooner rather than later.*

At about this time Colin Cutting suddenly and unexpectedly stepped down as clinical lead. This happened without any notice and despite the fact that all the clinical lead positions were due to be 'refreshed' in just a few months' time. There was much dismay and speculation within the department as to what had happened. Additionally, Mr Jain was suddenly suspended, presumably for his role in the two stent cases detailed above.

With Colin having resigned there was intense discussion about who would take over as clinical lead. Approached by a number of departmental members ranging from the secretarial staff and nursing staff to other surgeons, I didn't feel that I could take the job on, based as I was in FGH (RLI is the busier hospital) and with the sheer amount of hostility being directed towards me. However, Mr John Dickinson (associate specialist at RLI) was interested and after discussion we agreed to apply as a 'joint package' for the post. Within my full application I stated:

Discipline is the greatest problem of all in the department. A lack of this manifests itself in various different ways and has put the department in a very difficult position at the moment, with bullying and abusive behaviour, laziness and poor punctuality, unauthorised absences, low clinical standards, greed, misogyny and dishonesty all occurring on a frequent basis. These damaging, dysfunctional behaviours need to be excluded from the daily routines of the department and the department restored to the uniformly high clinical and professional standards that the Trust and the patients have a right to expect. It is therefore essential that the new clinical lead(s) immediately take steps to begin to eliminate such behaviour. Such behavioural traits are deeply embedded within the department and therefore by far the most important requirement of any successful clinical lead will be the unqualified commitment of the senior management and senior clinicians in excluding such behaviour. It is

*inevitable that attempts to clean up the department will be repeated-
ly challenged and the new lead(s) will need powerful and consistent
support in meeting this aspiration, possibly even requiring senior
management to approach external regulatory bodies for disciplinary
support.*

*It is also vital that the new lead(s) strike the right balance by
dealing with any future ill-discipline in a robust but also scrupu-
lously fair and honest fashion and do not allow their own behaviour
to deviate from the highest of professional standards. It is only by
imposing and retaining consistently fair and high standards that the
department will be able to sort out the issues above and look to
recruit and retain good quality staff in the future.*

After interview Mr Dickinson and I were subsequently given the
interim clinical lead job in early November, ahead of Mr Jain and Mr
Madhra who had also applied and, for this month, my missing AAS
payments of £1000 a week were restored (although October remained
unsettled).

Mr Jain was suddenly reinstated, sometime in late November
2015. I was told from several sources that this was after considerable
pressure from BAPIO (British Association of Physicians of Indian
Origin) and their legal arm, the Medical Defence Shield. After his
return to work meeting I was warned that he was seething, 'spitting
blood' and had vowed revenge over the protected disclosures that
had led to his suspension.

There was also an attempt to ambush me via the clinical incident
system by Messrs Jain and Naseem, with Ameeta Joshi concluding
that *the statement by AJ is therefore untrue.* However, no action was
taken over what now seems to have been a rather clumsy attempt at
reverse whistle-blowing.

At around this time I also learned that HM Coroner, Ms Hammond, had rejected the RCA report into the avoidable death from
neglect and was threatening at least one Regulation 28 against the
Trust.

A Regulation 28 is known as a report to prevent future deaths and flags up a Coroners concern about an ongoing risk to patients or members of the public. It is defined as follows:

> The Coroner has a legal power and duty to write a report follow-ing an inquest if it appears there is a risk of other deaths occurring in similar circumstances. This is known as a 'report under regula-tion 28' or a Preventing Future Deaths report because the power comes from regulation 28 of the Coroners (Inquests) Regulations 2013. The report is sent to the people or organisations, being in a position to take action to reduce the risk. They then must reply within 56 days to say what action they plan to take.

I was warned that the news was not at all well received by the Trust or the Critical Care Division, especially as a list of existing Regulation 28 reports is nationally available and is scrutinised by the regulators like the CQC and NHS England.

Having been appointed as joint interim clinical lead together with John Dickinson, we both felt that we needed to take a really firm stance over clinical standards and in late November I reported two further infected obstructed kidney cases that had been, in my opinion, negligently managed.

I initially reported them anonymously as I was so fearful of the inevitable backlash, but one of the senior managers clearly guessed that it was me and emailed me to ask me to formally report them in my name. I replied on the 15th December:

> Thanks ...,
>
> Yes, confidentially, it was me. You'll appreciate that one of the consultants involved has in the past stated that he 'wants to teach me a lesson' and the other has backed me up against a wall and threatened me with 'serious trouble' in the event of further clinical incident reports, so I really do have to remain anonymous. I was hoping that the division would pick these cases up without a CI, but Ameeta told me to formally submit them. Both seem to have been genuine incidents, both have documented obstructed kidneys, both

were clearly septic and both should have been stented just as soon as possible.

I am left utterly disbelieving of this situation where, with a Coroners Regulation 28 hanging over us and Ameeta threatening a GMC referral in the event of further inadequately treated infected obstructed kidneys, we have had two further cases treated with such a lack of urgency.

There is another case too, but as this precedes Ameeta's letter regarding mandatory safe management of these cases, I'll let that one go past.

I can't overemphasise the importance of keeping my name anonymous, and it's worth bearing in mind the fact that the individual who tipped me off about these cases was not prepared to submit CI's, presumably fearful of the consequences,

Peter.

Again, these two cases grossly violated the Royal College of Surgeons standard of three hours to intervention. One patient took about eight days to get to surgery, the other was discharged home on antibiotics without any surgery at all, before being readmitted and operated on as an emergency by Mr Dickinson, our associate specialist several days later.

Once again, there was no feedback whatsoever.

Shortly after submitting the email I was very dismayed to hear that Ms Hammond, the Coroner who had originally rejected the RCA report into the avoidable death patient had gone on long term sick leave. Her colleague, perhaps not fully aware of the circumstances, had apparently withdrawn the threat of a Regulation 28 and had closed the case.

This seemed like a very ominous development for me. Having vigorously flagged up my concerns about the potential for future deaths myself, I had hoped for robust support from the Coroner and the Coroner's office, especially as the Coroner had given me a clear instruction during the inquest.

Compounding my fears and despite numerous conversations with my contact at the CQC, the regulator seemed to be more minded to believe the assurances provided by the Trust that things were 'in hand', that there had been no disobedience to the Coroner and that appropriate investigations and measures had been taken. With the CQC leaning towards the Trust's bland reassurances, my ongoing £1,000 a week pay cut (resumed in December 2015) and the withdrawal of the Coroner's office from scrutiny of the ongoing clinical quality issues in the department, I felt extremely exposed. Although I continued to receive a lot of quiet and unofficial support from within and outside the department, no one else was openly prepared to speak up or approach one of the regulators, facing what appeared to me to be a concerted campaign to cover over the issues.

We also had ongoing personal behavioural problems at the time, with several incidents over inappropriate behaviour at consultant level. Offensive comments were variously made about a homosexual patient, Muslims, white women and a young homeless man, with several female members of the department being reduced to tears by aggressive and demeaning attitudes and comments.

As a consequence, I made a point of going through the NHS Behavioural Standards Framework on at least two occasions with the department, pointing out that offensive and prejudiced comments directed at the personal characteristics of staff and patients were entirely unacceptable.

UNFORTUNATELY, MY APPOINTMENT as joint clinical lead seemed to result in an almost immediate backlash, with both Mr Naseem and Mr Jain submitting grievances about me within days of my appointment, Mr Naseem on 23rd November and Mr Jain on 30th November.

Mr Naseem's grievance was about being asked to improve his punctuality. He had regularly arrived significantly late for a joint clinic going back many, many months, repeatedly throwing the clinics out of time. This delayed both patients and staff and on some occasions required another surgeon (Mr Mohammed Saqib) to turn in for work on his morning off to compensate and other staff to work through their lunch breaks. At our first departmental meeting, Mr

Dickinson and I made a generic plea (being very careful not to mention any names) for staff to start turning up on time for their joint commitments. Mr Naseem then turned up just under an hour late at the very next joint clinic and accused me of bullying and abusing him after I had politely asked him to start turning up on time.

At the same departmental meeting, John Dickinson and I had also emphasised, again without mentioning names, the importance of consultants taking personal clinical responsibility for sick patients during their on-call shift. On his very next on-call weekend, Mr Jain phoned me up on a Saturday evening (when I was starting a week of annual leave and was asleep in bed), demanding that I take personal clinical responsibility for a sick patient of his that required emergency surgery. He had made it clear that he didn't want any responsibility for the patient, instead wanting me to go into the hospital and document my assuming of responsibility in the notes. He also hinted that he wanted me to carry out the surgery. I politely declined, pointing out equally politely but firmly that clinical responsibility under these circumstances rested with the admitting surgical consultant on-call and not with the clinical lead. Mr Jain then proceeded in his grievance to accuse me of bullying and abusive behaviour in strikingly similar language to that of Mr Naseem's grievance.

I was never shown the written grievances at the time but simply had parts of them read out to me in a meeting with HR several months later.

To my sheer disbelief, it was only when these grievances and the transcripts were declared a few weeks prior to the Tribunal hearing in 2018 that I realised that, in addition to the written accusations of bullying and abusive behaviour, both Mr Jain and Mr Naseem also appeared to imply acts of racism by myself. These had clearly then been copied around both the Critical Care Division and the Human Resources department and quite possibly, outside the Trust.

At the end of the month (December 2015) my overtime payments were cut again by the Critical Care Division and never restored, despite me continuing to work the extra sessions and despite numerous verbal and written protests. The other consultants in the department continued to be paid the full rate of £500 per session for their extra AAS sessions and were still getting paid at this rate long after I had finally been forced into resignation.

————————

MY VALIDATION WORK, aiming to discharge the unnecessary follow-up patients, was still ongoing in late 2015. I had a fair bit of most Tuesdays as 'flexible time' to cover this work and it was clearly starting to reveal more than was intended about the division's finances and governance. It was clear to me that dozens, if not hundreds of thousands of pounds of precious NHS funding had been squandered on unnecessary premium rate (AAS) urology clinics, with needless follow-up appointments resulting in the continuous and unnecessary recirculating of patients who could and should have been discharged.

Over the previous two to three years, whenever I had found one of the more extreme examples of a patient that I felt was being followed up inappropriately, I wrote to the patient, explaining the logic of their discharge and copied the letter through to Belinda, my line manager at that time as well as the GP. By this point, Belinda's file had built up into a very sizeable and heavy lever arch file, full of hard evidence of unnecessary follow-ups, a very significant number having been repeatedly followed up through AAS 'premium-rate' clinics.

I had thought that the Critical Care Division would have been grateful for my efforts in discharging large numbers of unnecessary follow-ups and reducing their huge spend on unneeded AAS clinics, but as time went on it become clear to me that my success in reducing unnecessary follow-up numbers had become an embarrassment.

A table showing the effects of my efforts in reducing the numbers of urology department patients breaching on their waiting time targets during 2015 is below, beginning with my appointment at FGH in April 2015 when I had more time to do this work. Different categories of the numbers of patients breaching on their targets for follow-up are displayed. Table 6 is worst breaches, table 5 intermediate and table 1 is the least urgent category. The X axis is the time from April 2015 (just after I'd been appointed to FGH) to about October 2015. The table was presented to the Employment Tribunal in 2018.

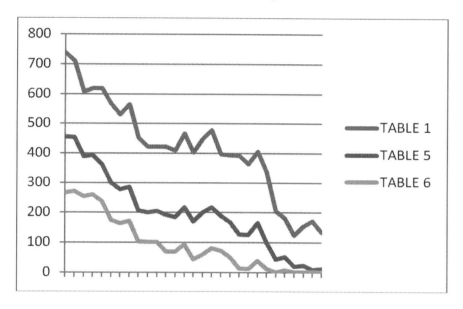

The impact of my validations (which at this point I was largely doing during my Tuesday flexible sessions or in my evening or weekend spare time) was commented upon in each of the divisional meetings that I attended. There was speculation about whether such inefficiencies and wastage of funds might be going on in other departments and I believe that attempts were made to expand the exercise to other specialities. It clearly was an awkward subject for the division as it implied massive inefficiency. I sensed a distinct back-pedalling on my work, with complaints that I wasn't doing (much less efficient) formal clinics or operating lists at the expense of devoting my Tuesday flexible time to discharging all these patients.

Not only did my validation exercise and its conclusions attract some serious criticism from a small number of colleagues, but it was at about this point that someone broke into and carefully searched

Belinda's private office. Despite the office being locked, access was clearly gained, the only item taken being the large lever arch file of evidence of unnecessary follow-ups. This simply vanished, together with all the evidence contained within it. It was never seen again and I suspect that it was shredded.

At around this time it appears that a further secretive attempt was made to get me into trouble, with Mr Jain circulating an email claiming that I'd been carrying out private work whilst claiming NHS sick pay during my first episode of ventricular ectopics way back in about 2012. These small, once-weekly clinics, carried out in my NHS free time had, of course, been approved by Belinda as a part of my phased return to work plan towards the end of my sick leave and documented as such. Additionally, my requests to return to NHS work had been turned down until I'd been cleared by the cardiologists. Mr Jain was well aware of both of these facts, but it didn't stop him from copying his complaints to the Trust's whistle-blowing guardian and whistle-blowing non-executive director. Astonishingly, the email also contained historical photocopied details of the patients attending my small private clinic from 2012 and the responses referred to other conversations about me of which I still remain in ignorance. Clearly, Mr Jain had been covertly collecting information on me for years. Once again, it seemed like a clumsy attempt at reverse whistle-blowing and once again I was given no chance whatsoever to respond, being completely unaware of these goings-on until the email and details were declared in the legal bundle of evidence in early 2018.

CHAPTER THIRTEEN

Detriment, demotion and the beginning of the end

IN EARLY JANUARY 2016 we had a departmental inspection by the Royal College of Surgeons. Hopeful that this might at least validate my and other clinicians concerns, to my disappointment the visiting team seemed anxious to steer conversation away from the specific clinical errors and incidents of retaliation and were clearly more comfortable with neutral and generic discussions about a 'dysfunctional department' and 'handover'. Also, they were rather embarrassingly unaware of some of the incidents that I had reported but which obviously hadn't been passed on to them.

Nevertheless, the visiting team from the Royal College were clearly uncomfortable about some of the issues around clinical standards in the department particularly with respect to emergencies and the treatment of urological sepsis. Despite the language in the report being rather anodyne and non-specific, it was clear that they acknowledged my concerns regarding clinical standards. Particular mention was made of the avoidable death and Coroner's case involving Mr Jain and Mr Naseem in 2015, with the Royal College commenting on their concerns over both the clinical management of the case and the risks of a repeat incident. Comment was also made about the poor quality and documentation of the Morbidity and Mortality meetings, where the Patient A cover-up had, of course, taken place.

During my discussions with the Royal College I was told that whilst they'd had extremely good feedback in general about my and Mr Dickinson's clinical leadership, it had also been alleged by a very small number of people that having me as the joint clinical lead was racist. I was warned that this would undoubtedly hamper my chances of continuing my role as joint lead clinician when it was renewed in February 2016.

I continued to feel considerable hostility towards myself from Mr Jain and Mr Naseem following the Royal College inspection and up to the point of the formal and definitive clinical lead interviews. Mr Madhra was supposed to be on a return to work scheme but was barely ever seen in the hospital, routinely failing to attend his supervised clinics and operating lists. Despite no doubt receiving his full contractual entitlement to salary plus on-call allowance, he seemed to be simply refusing to work. He finally left the Trust by 'mutual arrangement' in late 2018.

Encouraged by the strong support of the twenty or so regular members of the urology department, John Dickinson and I re-applied jointly for the lead job, once again emphasising our commitment to high personal and professional standards of behaviour. We then learned that both Mr Jain and Mr Naseem had stood against us. There was much dismay from the wider department and much trepidation from both Mr Dickinson and myself, particularly as I was still the subject of the ongoing grievances. I'd originally dismissed these as laughable and ridiculous, but now it seemed obvious to me that they had been timed tactically to damage my re-application.

After a lot of agonising, John and I agreed to stand down. I was particularly mindful at this point of the warning from the Royal College of Surgeons and felt that to stand against Mr Naseem and Mr Jain and to lose would be the worst of all possible worlds.

Both John and I came under much pressure from the wider department to reconsider our positions.

A close colleague emailed me simply saying: *This is a shame....* I replied on 22nd February:

> *It's a disaster, personally and for the Dep't (I think) but I can't face the retribution and abuse that is inevitably heading my way now. The best way to minimise it is to step down.*

I recall us both receiving several phone calls from senior managers and clinicians exhorting us to stand and also had emails and phone calls requesting and incentivising us to reapply from both Dr Walker and Ms Joshi.

In the end, John and I gave in to immense pressure and agreed to stand again as a joint package.

The interview went very smoothly and positively and I really didn't feel that I could have done any better, even being able to repeat the rather clunky definition of clinical governance and the ten clinical standards as laid out by Sir Bruce Keogh (previously National Medical Director for NHS England)! I was pretty sure that none of the other candidates would have prepared as thoroughly.

Late afternoon on the day that we were due to hear the result, I 'phoned John Dickinson to ask if he'd heard anything. I was met with a deafening silence.

He then asked, 'Haven't you been told?!!' He went on to explain that he and Mr Naseem had been offered the job jointly at around lunchtime. He had turned this down and the job had been given to Mr Naseem alone.

I received no call that day or evening. I lay awake all night, wondering what was going on and how I could possibly keep my job, now that the person who had delivered the phone call responsible for finally driving me out of Lancaster and who was jointly responsible for disobeying the Coroner over the death of Mr A, for other clinical errors and for the Royal Colleges concerns over the poor quality M&M meetings was now my direct superior. Despite having an outstanding grievance and, in my opinion, a clear grudge against me, he would now be responsible for my job plan, pay, hours of work, holidays, terms and conditions etc.

I had a meeting with Mr George Nasmyth (Associate Medical Director) the following morning. He seemed surprised that I still hadn't been told the result, telling me that 'It was because you were judged to be un-appointable as a result of the grievances submitted against you.' I replied that the grievances were ridiculous, fake and had clearly been timed tactically to damage my application by the very two people who had applied against me. He shrugged. I went on to describe how I felt now that one of the people who had run me out of Lancaster had been made clinical lead and described my feelings about the previous cover-up and misleading of the Coroner. 'I'll urgently email David (Walker),' he told me, turned his back and started typing. I never got to see that email and it was never declared in the evidence to the Tribunal despite a number of requests.

Immediately after that meeting I was asked to go to meet Human Resources for the formal investigation into the two grievances from Mr Jain and Mr Naseem. I wasn't made fully aware at that time of the fact that both grievances had again raised the issue of racism. I robustly defended my position and was informed at a later date by Louise Slee (line manager) that I had no case to answer. Thankfully, as far as I am aware Mr Jain took the matter no further and his complaint appears to have ended there. Mr Naseem, however, having been informed of the conclusions of the investigation told the Trust that he wanted to take it further and that he would be speaking with Morecambe Bay's respect champion. I never found out how much further this went although I was made aware at a later date by Louise of the fact he had gone outside the organisation for support.

That evening I finally got a phone call from Dr David Walker, well over 24 hours after the other candidates had been informed. There was no explanation or apology for the pressure that he and others had put me under to stand against my better judgement and he seemed entirely disinterested in what was now an impossible position for me, bluntly telling me that Mr Naseem had interviewed better than me. He seemed entirely dismissive of the fact that it had been Mr Naseem's phone call that had precipitated my resignation from the RLI and also told me that Ms Joshi had been very strongly in favour of appointing Mr Naseem despite the pressure that she had also put on me to stand against my better judgement. He went on to inform me that the executive felt that Mr Naseem was a better doctor and clinician, better manager and set a better example to the department than myself and that he would provide me with a list of those qualities where he and the executive had judged me to be inferior.

I felt utterly utterly crushed.

After another near sleepless night I sent an email at 4.50am on 9th March 2016, copying it to the other members of the interview panel.

Dear David and Ameeta,

I am writing to express my very real anxiety, distress and disbelief over the appointment of Mr Naseem as clinical lead.

I haven't yet slept tonight, nor did I sleep last night as a result of firstly the anticipation and now the reality of the appointment. To be told that Mr Naseem is a better role model and clinical leader than myself for the department is a crushing insult and sad and shocking reflection of senior clinicians opinion of my own commitment and standards. I also think it was deeply inappropriate, considering my anxieties below, to keep me waiting for 9 days for an answer and well over 24 hours after the successful candidates were notified.

During my 15 year spell in the Trust I believe that I have at all times worked hard and diligently, arriving on time, filling my sessions as much as possible, working extra sessions without remuneration and over the last 12 months transforming the quality of urological clinical care at FGH following my being forced out of Lancaster. I have built strong and healthy relationships with patients and staff at all levels and have encouraged all to follow my clinical standards and leadership. I have spent considerable time (inc significant evening and weekend time) carrying out many hundreds, probably thousands of patient validations over the last year, thus saving the Trust many dozens of thousands of pounds in potential waiting list initiatives and fines. During my brief tenure as joint interim clinical lead I have built healthy and helpful relationships with general surgical and medical colleagues at FGH as well as with my management colleagues....

I withdrew from the applications for the definitive lead job as I was fearful (as laid out in previous conversations and emails) of the backlash and intimidation that might result from my standing against Mr N and Mr J. Having been forced out of my previous post at Lancaster and having been on the verge of resigning, just under a year ago I was particularly mindful of the recent malicious clinical incidents and grievances submitted by both of these individuals, the potential for these attacks to intensify and the fact that these might (as they were probably intended to) hinder my application.

I feel that it was very wrong for you both to pressure me into standing against Mr N and Mr J against my better judgement. I was given the impression that I was a strong candidate and that both of you wished to see me continue with the hard work and commitment that I had exhibited alongside John Dickinson in the definitive role. Clearly this was not the case and I now find myself in the worst of all possible worlds, having run for the job, under pressure from yourselves and with, I believe, the hopes and expectations of a large majority of the wider department behind me and having been summarily rejected. It is a crushing and very public humiliation to be told, as I was this evening and after waiting so long, that Mr N sets a better example for the department and that the Trust has more confidence in his leadership abilities and standards than in my own.

I went on to say…

I have pushed tirelessly for the prompt management of urological emergencies…. My theatre utilisation figures (mentioned in the RCS report) demonstrate the huge excess of emergency workload that I have carried for the Dep't over the years and the lack of engagement of several of my colleagues in such work. I have tirelessly flagged up clinical errors and medical/surgical failings over the years, initially informally and more recently via the clinical incident system as standards have fallen further and further within the Dep't. I would have hoped that an individual with such qualities would have been recognised and rewarded.

I have already paid a heavy price for my commitment to high standards and refusal to ignore clinical failings, having to endure constant hostility from colleagues…, falsified clinical incidents and faked up grievances, veiled threats and attempts to unsettle and upset me including, astonishingly, a successful attempt by Mr N a couple of years ago to disrupt a long-planned family holiday. I have been falsely reported to the police as a racist and someone in the

Dep't triggered a faked-up stream one GMC enquiry against me, lasting six months. It was an abusive phone call from Mr N which ended my career at Lancaster and, whilst he did later apologise (under pressure) this would have triggered my resignation from the Trust had I not hurriedly been found an alternative post in Barrow. I therefore have absolute confidence that Mr N will once again sooner or later indulge in attempts to unsettle and unseat me from the Trust now that the executive have endowed him with the reach to do so and I have no confidence in my ability to continue to survive such attacks, or the ability of the Trust to support and protect me.

I will take some time over the forthcoming days to reflect on my position. My wider family are all firmly of the opinion that the above events have made my position untenable and that I should resign and are desperately worried about my health and ability to continue to endure this job.

I hope that I have made my position clear and, as we discussed, I'd appreciate a list of all those qualities where the executive felt that Mr Naseem's clinical, managerial and people skills exceed my own.

Yours sincerely,
Peter Duffy.

Of course and as usual there was no acknowledgement or response from any of the recipients. Nor did I ever receive the list of all those qualities where the Trust's executive felt that Mr Naseem's clinical, managerial and people skills exceeded my own (as Dr Walker had promised).

I then emailed Ms Joshi again on 11th of March saying:

Dear Ameeta,

I know that you've been away and probably have a pile of emails to get through but I'd be really grateful for your reaction to events earlier this week as laid out below.

I'm still desperately upset about this and have heard precisely nothing back from any of the original recipients. I emailed F and AG and similarly have had no response or acknowledgement. Struggling to get any sleep and the only real relief that I've had was yesterday's list which was so busy that I actually forgot about these issues for a few hours.

I feel that I've gone from a situation where I was content, secure and enjoying my job to a situation where I have no sense of security whatsoever. As below, it really isn't a sustainable situation, even for a few weeks as I'm already exhausted. I'll book leave for 6/52 but not sure I'll last that far,

Peter.

Ms Joshi phoned me back a day or two later, but I got little sympathy and was repeatedly told 'Look, you're a good clinician,' which didn't really do anything to allay my anxieties about being driven out of the Trust.

From this point on I submitted no more formal written clinical incidents whilst in the employment of the NHS, although overall clinical and behavioural standards remained depressingly the same. There was a mixture of sympathy, outrage and disbelief from the department over the way that the appointment had been made and the way that I had been treated and a real sense of foreboding as to what the future held, both for me and the department as a whole.

Throughout this period I remained in close, probably weekly contact with the CQC by telephone. However, whilst my contact there seemed concerned and listened carefully to my increasing worries and was, I believed, escalating these within the CQC, it seemed clear that the CQC's senior managers preferred the Trust's version of events, namely that these issues were historical and had been addressed, with no ongoing risks to patients.

My pay cut of £1000 a week continued despite my protests and there seemed to be a determined attempt going on by the Critical Care Division in particular to undermine me, portray me as a liability and make the job undoable. Only in the build up to the Tribunal hearing was it revealed that 'highly important' and 'confidential' emails were being covertly circulated about me during this period, accusing me of losing the division over £100,000 per year in non-productivity and inappropriate invoicing, with talk of investigations and enquiries. Needless to say, I had no chance to repudiate these lies as, like so many other things, they were kept entirely secret, only coming to light in the weeks leading up to my Tribunal hearing.

Ironically, it was at this time that the front-line staff of UHMB's organisation voted me their 'Doctor of the Year'. The nominations had been collected for a good number of weeks or months earlier and I had no idea that anything was going on until Dr Bari, Associate Medical Director, stopped me in the hospital car park to congratulate me on the number and quality of nominations from the Trust's other employees some weeks before the award took place.

Furness General Hospital:
FGH Consultant Urologist wins 'Doctor of the Year' award

> *The 'Doctor of the Year' award celebrates doctors who continuously go 'that extra mile', showing strong leadership and professionalism.*
>
> *Mr Peter Duffy, Consultant Urologist at FGH, moved to Barrow a year ago and streamlined the care of the urology patients at FGH, bringing waiting lists down to a level that had not been seen for a considerable time prior to his arrival. Peter was praised for treating all members of the team equally – getting stuck in – even mopping the floor between theatre cases!*

The overwhelming endorsement of the front-line staff seemed to make no difference whatsoever to management attitudes to me and we subsequently had a Departmental meeting in April attended by Dr Walker, Ms Joshi and Ms Ellison, a senior manager from Critical Care Division and the person who was alleged to have pushed through my £10,000 a year pay cut back in 2010.

The body language was very hostile towards me. I found myself seated at the bottom end of the table with Dr Walker, Ms Ellison, Ms Joshi, Mr Naseem and Mr Jain all sitting together at the top end from where the presentations are given. As if to further emphasise my demotion and deep unpopularity with senior management, it was here in front of the whole extended department that a totally unexpected statement was made about moving my base hospital from RLI to FGH.

By the way Peter, we'll be moving your base hospital to Barrow now....

The statement was made first by Ms Joshi and referred directly to me by name. Worse still, the threat was then reiterated by Ms Ellison after Ms Joshi had left the room to answer a mobile call. On the second occasion I pointed out that UHMB's rule was that consultants had to live within 30 minutes' drive of their base Hospital. Moving my base to FGH would put me a minimum of 75 minutes away. Sue replied by saying:

Ah ha Peter. We've checked up on you. You don't get paid to do any emergencies or on-call work so we think that we can move your base anyway....

Forcibly moving my base hospital to FGH would have made my job utterly untenable (even without everything else that was going on). It is an NHS rule that travel to your base hospital isn't recognised as work (even if it is 2½ hours and 90-odd miles of driving per day as was my case), nor does the NHS employee get travel costs to their base hospital. Additionally, I'd only ended up at FGH because of the bullying and abusive behaviour at Lancaster. By unilaterally changing the agreement that had taken me to FGH and that still applied to everyone else in the department, the division would have rewritten my contract and timetable at a stroke, removing 2½ hours a day of work related travel from my remuneration (totalling ten hours a week, about 20% of my basic pay). This was, of course, on top of the ongoing deduction of £1,000 per week from my overtime pay. The change would also have meant that, uniquely amongst the consultant body, I would have to use my own car for commuting across the Trust (400 to 500 miles per week) and pay all expenses and depreciation as opposed to the other consultants and senior managers who were either using lease cars or receiving mileage allowances.

Ms Joshi later denied there was any intention to do this when I met with her in October 2016, but in the subsequent legal filings to the Tribunal the Trust clearly stated that the Critical Care Division *required the Claimant to relocate his base hospital....* completely contradicting her denial and confirming the division's intent.

At the same meeting we were all given jobs to do as a consequence of the Royal College recommendations. I felt that I had been given a very disproportionate amount of work (especially as I had by far and away the most arduous timetable) and felt that once again that I was being singled out for punishment. The CQC reviewed these actions the following month and in one of my telephone conversations, my contact commented that the CQC team had speculated about this large excess of work over and above my regular commitments and whether I was being *set up to fail.*

It was at this point that the department staff at large concluded that there was a determined push going on to make my life impossible and thus expel me from the Trust. After the prolonged and very tense meeting with David Walker, Sue Ellison and Ameeta Joshi, about six people gathered round me to express their extreme unease over what they had just witnessed, their disbelief over the hostility that had been shown to me, the sense that the division wanted these issues closed down at any cost and had *got it in for me* and their belief that my position was being undermined and made untenable. As I testified to the Tribunal, a close, long term colleague quietly commented, 'You've made enemies here... they've got the means, the motive and now with Saleem as lead, the opportunity to finally get shot of you...'

The strength of belief that I was being deliberately forced out was such that at the next departmental meeting, we openly debated the likelihood of my forced resignation or dismissal. Mr Naseem as the new clinical lead announced that he intended to review and revise everyone's job plans, a very extensive exercise and one that would cause considerable work and disruption for everyone, as well as, of course, giving the division the opportunity to follow through with their threat to switch my base hospital to the other end of the Trust. It was pointed out to Mr Naseem by another consultant that there was little point in wasting large amounts of departmental time on such an exercise in the face of the clear divisional intention to force me into resignation. If I were to be forced to resign then this would, of course, mean that there'd have to be yet another job planning exercise after I'd gone and that the first would have been a complete waste of time.

Looking back, it seems remarkable that we openly and candidly discussed the ongoing bullying and illegal attempts to unseat me from my job. Not one single person disputed what at that point had become obvious. There was widespread support for deferring any job planning exercise until it became clear as to whether the Division would succeed in dismissing me although Louise Slee, my line manager, approached me afterwards to point out that open discussions in official meetings of the attempts to force me into resignation was not exactly helping the department's morale!

Finally and after some debate, Mr Naseem acceded to the department's concerns and put off his job planning exercise, showing his irritation in a subsequent email to Ms Joshi, complaining about me and the discussions over my forced resignation delaying his intentions for job planning.

In the meantime I simply tried to cling on and submitted no further clinical incidents or concerns in the hope that somehow I might be allowed to hang on to my job at FGH (I'd repeatedly made it clear that under no circumstances did I feel it safe for me to return to the RLI). I continued to protest regularly over the ongoing £1000 a week cut in my AAS payments whilst everyone else continued to be paid the full rate for their regular AAS's.

Although I submitted no more clinical incidents during this period, on 21st April 2016 I was copied into an email string regarding the case of the potentially avoidable death of Mr A that had triggered the Coroner's intervention the previous year. The Associate Medical Director was retiring and clearly wanted to close the case down rather than pass it on to a successor. Fearful that the case would be closed down and covered up without HM Coroner's instructions being complied with, I didn't feel I could let this go past and, summoning up what little was left of my courage for one last stand, I replied, copying in the Medical Director and Clinical Director:

Hello ...,

I've been copied into this email string.

This is the Mr A case which is well known within the Dep't and which at one time seemed likely to trigger a coroners regulation 28. It was specifically flagged up by the very recent Royal College of Surgeons departmental review as the incident causing them the most concern, not least because of the risks of a further similar incident.

I have been very careful about whom I copy this email to, as the case has caused considerable controversy and ill-feeling within the department and the ramifications are far from being sorted out. My humble advice would be to pass this on to your successor, as I see no possibility of the case being closed down within the next few weeks, not least as we still have to comply with the Coroners instructions of a year ago to discuss the case in our morbidity and mortality meeting, something that a section of the department has so far refused to do.

There are a number of worrying threads to the case which I have repeatedly flagged up:

• A potentially avoidable patient death, as per the coroner's verdict.

• A tendency for some consultants to treat infected obstructed kidneys conservatively or casually, or without due attention to immediate emergency intervention as per national standards.

• Similar cases with one previous coroner's case avoidable death from inadequately treated renal sepsis at FGH and others where there has clearly been serious risk to life from delayed intervention, even after the (Patient A) case came to light.

• Successful attempts to suppress discussion of the case.

• Refusal to comply with the coroner's instructions and attempts to mislead the coroner via the individual consultant reports submitted last year.

• An internal enquiry which did not seem to address the critical issue of the lack of immediate emergency intervention on the Sunday or the following day despite the consultant microbiologist's recommendations (the Royal College of Surgeons Standard of Care is operative intervention within 3 hours of diagnosis. It took 48

hours to get Patient A to theatre and even then it was not the on-call surgeon that carried out the procedure).

• A dysfunctional department with bullying, intimidation, threats and resignations.

• A clique of senior individuals whose clinical practice in some cases varies greatly from accepted best practice.

• And of course we now have an external and impartial expert surgical authority expressing very significant concern about the case and about future risks to patients (the recent Royal College of Surgeons review).

The similarities with issues flagged up elsewhere in the Trust in the Kirkup report [The midwifery scandal] *won't have escaped your attention.*

*I would personally welcome an opportunity to clarify my own role in the case as I was very unhappy with some of the criticisms made of me in the original report and felt under pressure (both at the time of the inquest and subsequently) to throw the coroner off the scent. I have never had an opportunity to respond to these criticisms. I think the case **should** be discussed in our M&M meeting (esp' now that we have a new audit lead) but we will need a very senior presence to stop the meeting deteriorating into rancour and shouting, as has happened when major clinical incidents have been discussed in the past. I therefore feel, as above, that it would be best from your own point of view if the case were to be passed to your successor. My greatest fear is of a repeat incident (a fear shared by the Royal College of Surgeons) in which case, if the RCA is closed, I think that we could all be accused of having known about dangerous practice and having failed to act rigorously to protect patients from future risk.*

All the best and I hope that you have a long and happy retirement,

Peter

True to form, I had no response from any of the individuals copied in to the email, nor was the final report ever sent to me or made available to the Tribunal.

IN THE SAME MONTH I was requested to attend a meeting with David Walker and Ameeta Joshi. Smelling a particularly large rat, I queried the nature of the meeting and was told:

Hi Peter,

It's regarding the concerns you raised via email to them both.

Kind Regards,
Trust HQ PA: Medical Director

I wasn't so sure about this and neither was the wider department. A colleague sent a simple email saying *Oh dear Peter….*

The email implied that the meeting was to do with my own messages regarding the clinical lead and departmental issues (I hadn't done a recent joint email about anything else) but several colleagues urged me to either take a solicitor or British Medical Association representative. With the concerns in the department that my job was being made impossible, they were particularly worried that the meeting would result in further detriment, disciplinary action or even dismissal. In the end and thinking that it was a bit confrontational to take a legal or BMA person, I went on my own.

The meeting was nothing to do with my emails, but was about the two patients that Mr Jain had neglected to stent and had then (in the opinion of many of those present) misinformed the department about. I had not submitted any emails regarding these two patients from the previous year and therefore went in to the meeting entirely unprepared. It was clear that the meeting was accusatory but after standing up for myself I was finally and to my relief told that there would not be any disciplinary process.

The meeting at least gave me the opportunity to voice concerns about both the department and my treatment to date. I was determined to get my concerns across, particularly now that I felt that my vocation had been almost prised out of my grasp, telling my seniors:

As you know full well this is the latest in a very, very, very long line of, and I am choosing my words carefully, negligent actions that have gone on in the department that have had serious and sometimes lethal consequences and I don't feel like I can just sit by and watch these cases go through.

I went on to say:

Since then we have had things like the Patient A case. Again we are still in contempt of Court over that. We still haven't discussed it at the mortality meeting and Patient A died an eminently avoidable death because two people just couldn't be bothered to take him to theatre and the sad thing about it and the bit that I have a got a bad conscience about is that by that stage I had succeeded in being so intimidated that I didn't put a clinical incident in about it, and the Coroner picked me up on it because I felt I had been so beaten down to the point where all that came back from the clinical incidents was more... unpleasantness.

Going on, I stated:

This is being portrayed as a personality clash, dysfunctional individuals not getting on.

I told my seniors:

It is not, it's absolutely not about that, it's about whistle-blowing, clinical standards and it's about a small cohort of individuals who are not prepared to work to what you might call national minimum standards and who will get the boot into anyone who tries to sort that out.

I particularly expressed my worries about the misleading RCA report into the Patient A case, stating:

The Royal College flagged this up as being the case they were most concerned about and where they felt this was the greatest danger of it being repeated, whereas our own investigation... was... hopeless. They walked straight past the really big issue, the elephant in the room and they just didn't acknowledge it which was the lack of action when this man needed emergency surgery. The Coroner picked up on it and we were so lucky to get out from under a Coroner's regulation 28. Only because she went off sick we got away with that so this could have ended up very differently and I'm sorry to say it but the investigation… was not an adequate investigation and I think any external urologist that came and looked at that would have just gone… 'They set out to not find a problem.'

*We have had two more I would say negligently managed infected obstructed kidneys since the [Patient A] case, we got away with both of them and one of them again was appalling and we were very lucky to get away with that so habits have **not** changed.*

I went on to describe the effects on my own self-esteem and morale:

You know, I mean I nearly took my own life over that GMC enquiry I really did, I really did…. my wife's a GP and I knew what I was going to take [from her doctor's bag] and at what time I was going to take it so my boys didn't find me. I…. I don't think you have any idea what I've gone through in this job and I still have nightmares about some of the cases I've had to deal with.

Finally, I voiced my fears about a possible whistle-blower witch-hunt and counter-allegations including racism against me, stating:

It doesn't take too much imagination to see a really difficult scenario emerging where other employees put in a fairly convincing complaint or grievance or incident or something and then I have no doubt the two of you would say that we would support you to the hilt, but ultimately it will land in the lap of somebody at the Trust's Solicitors and they will look at it and say 'you're not going to win this.' You can either, spend a six figure sum and lose, or you can get rid of him now and I suspect the two of you will do the right thing for the Trust which will be to get rid of me.

In return, I was made to feel that I'd over-reacted and that, whilst such things might have happened in the past, they certainly wouldn't happen that way now.

In response to these comments on my feelings I replied:

> *I do, I do, I'm afraid.... I mean these kinds of allegations carry an awful lot of weight don't they and if you have two people corroborating each other's accounts it could get so nasty. This is the sort of thing that is keeping me awake at night.*

Of course, within six months of this statement I'd been illegally dismissed and was unemployed.

The responses to my concerns now come across as non-specific platitudes but at the time seemed to me like a pretty specific assurance that no such retaliatory allegations had occurred. With hindsight, I should have read more into the exact wording. But at the time and in the heat of the moment I reassured myself that Dr Walker and Ms Joshi had been given the opportunity to fully inform me if such allegations had been made and hadn't done so. Very foolishly, I therefore wrongly concluded that no such allegations had been made. Again, there are lessons here for anyone facing a similar situation.

After the meeting was over I drove back to the urology office at the RLI, only to my surprise finding about half a dozen departmental members waiting behind for me after work, asking 'Have you been sacked?' and 'Have they forced you to resign?'

I replied that I had survived... *just about*...

All the meantime the £1000 a week pay cut continued and I continued my protests, consulting a British Medical Association (BMA) legal representative who told me, 'This is absolutely appalling but hang on in there.' I continued to do the extra sessions that I was not being paid for on the assurance from my line manager Louise that, 'You're clearly doing the sessions and they're clearly marked in your job plan to be paid at AAS rates so they'll have to pay you eventually.'

Heather, the local Morecambe Bay NHS whistle-blower guardian, advised me to keep the BMA involved and told me that she'd escalate the issues to senior management.

In May 2016 and after discussions with the BMA I drew up a formal grievance, showing it to my manager Louise. It read:

FORMAL GRIEVANCE

Dear ...,

Thank you in advance for looking into this formal grievance against the surgery and Critical Care Division of the University Hospitals of Morecambe Bay NHS Trust. I have already repeatedly tried to resolve this by all informal means and have waited well over six months for a resolution. As this informal process has failed I would like to escalate this to a formal grievance.

In late March 2015 I was transferred to FGH from RLI to take up a new job plan. I had been informally discussing this with our urology management for some weeks beforehand but the situation was suddenly brought to a head by an unexpected and very unpleasant phone call from a consultant colleague. My initial reaction was to resign immediately, but instead I was persuaded to remain in the Trust and transfer immediately to FGH....

....I think that it is very wrong that a decision then seems to have been taken by a person or persons unknown to substantially alter my contract and reduce my agreed salary package without discussion with me, resulting in the above shortfall. It is also wrong and wholly inappropriate for a series of vague reassurances to have been offered, resulting in my continuing to work 60+ hours a week for 48 hours of pay. Both the BMA and I consider this to be a case of a continuous unlawful deduction of wages which has resulted in my working of 60+ hours a week for a pay package that had covertly been reduced to 48 hours (12 PAs) [a PA is four hours work] *for the better part of a year.*

Finally, I understand that an alternative job plan has very recently been circulated showing my base hospital to be FGH and with DCC [direct clinical care] *time changed to SPA* [supporting professional activity] *time. This is emphatically not something that I agreed to or was even aware of and, again, I believe this to constitute quite a serious breach of standards and against your Job Planning Policy.*

Overall, I believe these events to be a very serious breach of contract and trust by my employer. I believe that employment law has been violated and I'd be grateful if these events could be urgently investigated and the appropriate action taken to correct this shortfall and to ensure that such a situation does not happen again.

Thank you in advance,
Peter Duffy.

I followed this up with some more pleadings for action and email exchanges in early June but did not hear anything definitive back. At around this point, to my despair, I was also told that Mr Naseem was still pursuing his grievance against me for asking him to turn up on time for joint clinics and had now gone outside the organisation with his grievance.

CHAPTER FOURTEEN

Shoot the messenger

EARLY SUMMER OF 2016 was distinguished for me by a dread and constant sense of incipient disaster.

By now, no one in the department was in any doubt that I was, in career terms, living on borrowed time. There was a palpable feeling of the members of the department waiting with bated breath for the event that would finally push me beyond my breaking point.

That point arrived on 15ᵗʰ June 2016. It was the long awaited (nine months) response from the Critical Care Division to my request and grievances, regarding payment of the ongoing issue of the missing £1,000 a week AAS earnings.

The document itself was titled as a 'Job Plan Review'; an ominous opening gambit as I hadn't asked for a job plan review but had simply asked to be paid, like everyone else was getting paid, for the 15 hours or so of extra work that I was doing every week over and above my 48 hour working week. Whilst the document was accompanied by a pretty innocuous email, the contents of the Job Plan Review itself were a bombshell. The document seemed to me to be full of malicious inaccuracies and false accusations. It made it clear that the division had no intention of paying me for the vast majority of the AAS sessions that I had worked over the last nine months in good faith. It seemed clear (and indeed was also clear to the Tribunal panel some two years later) that the division was questioning my integrity by implying that I was not working sessions that I was claiming for, working part sessions when I was claiming for full sessions and was also alleging that I was claiming for sessions when I was already paid to be in the hospital anyway.

Scan-reading the document on Friday afternoon, I was immediately of the clear opinion that the Critical Care Division was implying fraud or attempted fraud by myself and equally clearly this made my position in the Trust and the NHS impossible. At this point I still hadn't spotted the sting in the tail which only became apparent to me over the following weekend. The Critical Care Division was threatening to go back through my previous NHS earnings 'recouping monies', a clear threat to punish me even further (the future 20% travel time pay cut on top of the £1,000 a week was still hanging over me). Even a brief calculation convinced me that the division seemed to be gearing up to come after me for at least a five figure sum in addition to the missing monies and of course the ongoing threat to change my base hospital.

It is still difficult to put into words how hurtful and offensive I found these accusations to be, particularly as I was clearly being singled out amongst all the consultants, but also because I felt that I was being accused of attempted fraud when in fact the exact opposite was true.

In fact, I had spent so very much of my time at UHMB working to try and increase the efficiency of the department, oppose wastage and eliminate what I considered to be financially sharp practice. Ironically, I was still doing the validation work at this point, much of it in my free evening and weekend time and still saving the division thousands of pounds per week despite the pay cut and the other punishments and detriments.

Nearly two years later, I was to describe my emotions at this point to the Employment Tribunal. Sitting at one of the secretaries desks with the offending report on the screen in front of me, I seemed to be looking down on the whole scene from the ceiling. Our middle grade doctor was telling me about a patient that he'd found complicated and challenging, but he might as well have been speaking to the wall. Numb and shocked to the core, it was clear that the Critical Care Division had finally succeeded in pushing me over the employment law cliff edge and I now had no choice but to resign.

As the Tribunal was to later describe it, *the final straw was a heavy one.*

On the same afternoon as the above wholly false and deeply offensive allegations I received another clinical incident aimed at myself by Mr Madhra. Despite hardly ever being seen in the hospital and having had nothing to do with this patient, he appeared to have accessed confidential patient information in order to submit the incident. The incident accused me of missing a major post-operative complication on a patient. However, I'd had nothing to do with the operation itself or the immediate post-operative care which had taken place 45 miles away at the RLI. Indeed, I had only seen the patient briefly, several weeks after the procedure, when she was moved to FGH before being discharged home. Furthermore, having been operated on at Lancaster, I wasn't even aware that the CT scan showing the complication (a clot in the main abdominal vein) even existed. Nevertheless, I was roundly blamed for not spotting and treating the complication.

After a sleepless weekend punctuated by runs of ventricular ectopics, I phoned in sick (I didn't even feel safe to drive, far less work). I was deeply intimidated by the threat of the Critical Care Division going back through my previous payments and 'recouping monies' as well as the still-outstanding threat to move my base hospital to FGH with a consequent 20% pay cut. My calculation was that they might end up demanding many dozens of thousands of pounds back from me and my family if they performed the same completely false accounting exercise that they had previously inflicted on other periods of my work. In addition to this I was facing a potential pay cut that that might slice another four figure sum per month off my already £1000 a week depleted earnings. I'd never heard of anything remotely close to such brutal, bullying and abusive treatment of an NHS employee. My sympathetic but helpless deputy line-manager made an appointment with occupational health and I made an appointment with my GP. Neither felt that there was any option for me other than to resign, my GP (married to an employment law solicitor), stopping me after a couple of minutes of my story, holding his hand up and telling me:

'My diagnosis it that you're being constructively dismissed.'

I informed the BMA by telephone who agreed with occupational health and my GP that my position had clearly been made entirely impossible and that I now had no choice but to resign. They advised me that I ought to try and work out my three month notice period as per GMC guidance rather than leave immediately. Sick to the core, well aware that I had no job to go to and having been bullied and beaten down into resigning from a vocation that I'd had since my teens, I drew up my resignation letter to David Walker the Medical Director which was sent on 6th July 2016. It stated:

Dear David,

I am writing to inform you that I am resigning from my position as consultant urological surgeon with immediate effect.

Please accept this letter as my formal notice and termination of my employment contract with the Trust.

I feel I have been left with no option but to leave. There are so many contributing factors to my decision including my physical and mental health, but the deciding issue has been the failure of the Trust to adhere to the salary and conditions which were agreed in March 2015 as a part of my revised job plan and transfer to FGH. Having persuaded me (as a result of the improved terms and conditions) to withdraw from applying for a job in Scotland in 2015, I believe that it was utterly wrong for the division to then block payment of the extra sessions that were agreed as part of the pay package. These extra sessions were to compensate me for the long and arduous hours including travel that the new FGH post would entail. Furthermore, I believe that the decision to stop paying the extra sessions (seemingly taken around the end of the year) should at the very least have been discussed and negotiated with me and preceded by a job planning meeting. It is entirely unacceptable that I was left working 60+ hours a week whilst being kept in the dark about the division's change of heart over my pay and conditions. It is also unacceptable that I should have to demand a grievance to find this out.

Additionally, part of my revised terms and conditions in 2015 were that the RLI would remain my base hospital so that I would retain the departmental lease car and costs and travel time from Lancaster to FGH would be included, just as they were when all the consultants took turns at covering FGH. At the last departmental meeting it was announced separately by both AJ and SE that the division will move my base hospital to FGH with a consequent loss of both travel time and the lease car. This directly contradicts the assurances that I was initially given in 2015, will further extend the gap between real hours worked and hours remunerated and will further reduce my income.

During my last week of work before becoming ill with a recurrence of my cardiac issues I received another malicious clinical incident aimed at myself and separately an email on 15th June, making it clear that, after an internal investigation the division will not abide by the agreed terms of my move to FGH in March 2015. The report stated that of the sessions that I was advised to claim, roughly a quarter were not worked, another quarter were done in time when I was already employed and the remainder were invoiced at the full sessional rate whilst only working part of it. The report even threatened to claw back monies that I have already earned. This was the last straw and I feel that these wholly unjustified assertions were designed to intimidate me and ruin any chance of rebuilding an already very fragile and badly damaged employee/employer relationship (see below).

On top of the recent events detailed above, I feel that I have been the long term recipient of much unwarranted and abusive behaviour from individuals employed by the Trust (both clinicians and managers) with this abuse stretching back many years. I believe the common factor to be my unswerving commitment to hard work and probity and my opposition to low standards and poor care, something which has made me vulnerable and which has not always gone down well with both managers and fellow clinicians. As you know, despite being quite a reserved and quiet individual with a marked aversion to conflict, I have spoken out on many occasions about some of the unsafe practices within the Trust with my concerns going back well over a decade. I believe that this commitment to high standards has in turn lead to many of the unpleasant outcomes that I have suffered. I do not feel that the Trust has supported me in this and feel that I have been treated very differently from other members of staff.

I cannot help but compare and contrast my own treatment with that of Mr Madhra, who seems to have been treated very deferentially despite his long track record of complaints and incidents. From a terms and conditions perspective he remains on full pay plus 20% plus on-call allowance despite the fact that he continues to refuse to turn up to work his weekly timetable and has failed to do so for many, many months now. He has, of course, not been clinically productive for something around 1/3 of his 16 years of employment in the Trust! I, on the other hand have diligently fulfilled my time-table and much more, yet seem to be have been targeted for a forced pay cut and adverse changes to my terms and conditions. It is diffi-cult to imagine two individuals being treated more differently and the sheer hypocrisy and double standards of this situation will sure-ly not have escaped you.

I believe that the Trust has violated employment law by breach of contract, illegal deduction of salary, failing to provide a safe working environment for me and by not treating me equitably. I feel that the Trust should have made strenuous efforts to protect me from manipulative and abusive behaviour and it was, of course, as a direct result of unchecked abusive behaviour that I initially devel-oped a stress related cardiac condition, something that put me on the coronary care unit during my first episode and that has dogged me over subsequent years and which has resulted in me currently being on sick leave.

I believe that the bond of trust that ought to exist between an employer and employee has been irretrievably broken with my health impaired as a result of the above actions and feel that the Trust has left me with no option other than to resign with immediate effect.

I am mindful of my obligations to the patients and, if my health recovers sufficiently then I will do my best to return and work out three months' notice to allow a successor to be appointed to FGH. However, this will of course be dependent on my feeling and being judged fit to practise, something that is certainly not the case cur-rently and I should make it clear that such an offer is purely an attempt to discharge my responsibilities to patient care and under no circumstances reflects any acceptance of the changes in my terms and conditions laid out in the email of June 15th, or the allegations contained within the email.

Please acknowledge receipt of this letter as soon as possible and I will do my best to ensure a smooth transition period until my leaving date.

Yours sincerely,
Peter Duffy.

I had hoped to receive an acknowledgement and a swift offer to meet, attend to my concerns and try to reverse the detriments and threats that had led to my resignation but nothing was received, not even an email or formal letter of acknowledgement. The vast majority of my colleagues both within and without the urology department were sympathetic but powerless to do anything to help. After several weeks of sick leave and returning from a thoroughly spoiled family holiday in Croatia that we had booked nearly a year earlier, I was invited to FGH for a return to work meeting.

I fully expected to be confronted or for the meeting to be 'gate-crashed' by someone from the Critical Care Division. But to my surprise and relief, no one intervened and the meeting was low key and sympathetic. The two very experienced managers expressed their disbelief about the dishonesty behind the statements made in the Job Plan Review document, their strong desire for me to return but also their helplessness in the face of the detriments and wholly false allegations made about me by more senior management.

I left the meeting with a sense of relief that at least I hadn't been accosted by anyone more senior and with the assurance that the accusations from the division would be strongly countered by the detailed inside knowledge of my workload and timetable displayed by the two managers in question.

There was a clear desire of the vast majority of the department, junior and middle management and allied specialities to see a concerted effort made to try and defuse the situation and to correct the entirely false accusations that had been made against me. However, it was already clear that senior management were determined to allow my resignation to run its course and to stay out of the way whilst my notice was worked out.

I restarted work the day after the return to work meeting on 3rd August 2016. I was excused operating out of fear that my cardiac issues would start up again. Despite this, I ended up operating on yet another mismanaged infected obstructed single kidney patient as an emergency during this spell. As I explained some three months later to Dr Walker and Ms Joshi:

'If there's anything more urgent than an infected obstructed kidney then it's an infected obstructed **single** kidney.'

Rather than undergoing immediate emergency surgery to relieve the obstruction and drain the infection, the patient in question had been sent to the Intensive Care Unit for antibiotics and haemofiltration, (a kind of dialysis to compensate for the blocked, infected and failing single kidney), rather than having their sepsis definitively treated and obstructed single kidney unblocked as would have been both logical and far, far safer.

Luckily the on-call ICU consultant at FGH the following day spotted the magnitude of the error, spoke to me and we were able to get the patient to theatre later the same day, about 24 hours after he should have been operated on. When I finally walked out of FGH for the very last time, he was doing well.

During my last few weeks several senior managers regularly brushed past me in the corridors without acknowledging me or looking me in the eye. On one of my very last days our Chief Executive of the time (now Dame Jackie Daniel), bumped into me outside ward 5 at FGH. She clearly recognised me (Fiona and I had sat next to her and chatted with her all evening at the 'Doctor of the Year' award to me just three to four months earlier). Nevertheless, she looked down at the ground and almost ran past me and down the corridor in her anxiety to get away from me.

I vividly recall watching her wobble away on her heels, thinking that she ought to wear more practical footwear on the wards and that she'd twist an ankle if she didn't slow down a bit. Knowing the background, the senior sister that I was with snorted and glanced across at me with raised eyebrows,

'My God, anyone would think you'd got Ebola virus...!'

Overall, there seemed to be a remarkable lack of regret or remorse from senior management over the fact that their current 'Doctor of the Year' had been forced into resignation under such awful circumstances.

It was, however, very noticeable during this period that I was left alone and hostile confrontations, emails, and fake clinical incidents ceased. Sadly, it felt very much like, having achieved their objective, it was now just a matter of a small number of colleagues and senior management keeping their heads down until my notice was worked out.

During this period, not one single individual from the executive was prepared to meet with me despite the intensive lobbying going on behind the scenes by loyal colleagues from both RLI and FGH.

I took considerable comfort from the fact that I got so many messages of anger, regret and disbelief from hospital friends and colleagues by email, cards and social media.

I'd hoped to continue with my vocation to work for and serve the patients of the North Lancashire and South Cumbria area at least until around 2025, but, after nearly 35 years I worked my last day for the NHS on 23rd August 2016.

We had a small farewell party, cards, food, gifts and quite a lot of tears in the urology office at FGH at the end of sixteen years of hard and committed work for UHMB (more than the then Chief Executive, Chair, Medical Director and Chief Operating Officer put together).

I was particularly moved by a small engraved glass presented to me by the Outpatient nurses and receptionists at FGH.

Peter Duffy
Simply the best
Missed by all
FGH outpatients

I still desperately miss each and every one of them too.

Not one single person from management or the executive turned up to wish me well.

At the other end of the Trust, Cath, my long-standing, loyal and outstanding RLI secretary organised a leaving card, collection and present for me. I'm ashamed to admit that it took many weeks for me to force myself to open the card and read it as I knew that there were comments of regret on the card from the very individuals who had caused me so much trouble, who had falsely accused me of racism and who had, I believed, been driving the process to get rid of me despite at least in part owing their jobs to me. The sense of hypocrisy and double standards left me utterly sickened and I deeply regret that I didn't show the gratitude to Cath that I should have done.

My last paid day after I'd taken my outstanding annual leave was 26th September. The meeting with senior management that had been repeatedly requested all the way back to early July by Colin, Belinda and others finally took place a few days later on 5th October.

This was, of course, the week after my employment had formally ceased and my first full week of joining the ranks of the unemployed.

Not one of us missed the significance of this timing, commented upon by all as being as obvious as a scream in the dark.

The meeting involved Dr Walker and Ms Joshi, Colin Cutting, Belinda Pharoah and an HR representative and covered a lot of ground, at last giving me an opportunity to vent my frustrations over the repeated failures of clinical standards, cover-ups and inadequate investigations in the department going back right to the beginning of my spell of employment in Morecambe Bay in 2000.

Even now, reading through the minutes makes my skin crawl. Not only was I now unemployed but I'd been forced to wait outside the Medical Director's office, in full view of a very large office full of secretaries, PAs and support staff like a naughty, humiliated schoolboy, waiting outside the Head's office to be told of his inexcusable behaviour and expulsion from school. Entering the Medical Director's room, I was faced with an array of people who only a few days earlier were colleagues but were now employed by an organisation that, it seemed, hated me sufficiently to see my vocation, reputation and finances and ultimately, family life destroyed. The sense of casual disinterest in my predicament from some just rubbed salt in the wound.

The meeting at least gave me a cathartic opportunity to get across my anger and frustration over the last nine months. Remarkably for someone who is usually very quiet and withdrawn, I spoke pretty passionately for what must have been a good five to ten minutes, talking through all the detriments and punishments from the Critical Care Division and the Trust as a whole. I covered the initial £1,000 a week pay cut, the seemingly stage managed demotion, the threat of moving my base hospital which would, of course, have involved another 20% pay cut as well as dumping 400 miles a week of commuting on me (in my own time and at my own cost, of course).

The final insult of the Job Plan Review was mentioned, together with the previous meeting where disciplinary action also featured:

'Ahh, I think being called in to see the two of you over Ash Jain's negligence with those two stent cases, I'm sorry, I think that was, out of order... I was told it was a meeting to discuss my concerns over the clinical lead issues and departmental standards and so on, so I was completely unprepared for that, and I think to have disciplinary action mentioned against me for simply exposing somebody else's lies and negligence was... preposterous, it was...surreal.'

The mention of this at last gave me an opportunity to make it totally and utterly clear that the accusations of false accounting laid at my door were entirely fictitious. As I put it:

'Then finally, finally, we need to move on to this document here. Sorry, I struggle to call it a document; it's more a malicious, malignant piece of fantasy fiction... OK, review of job plan. Now this was the thing that finally, I mean, it just made my resignation inevitable... I couldn't believe this.... I didn't ask for a review of job plan, I simply asked what had happened to the money that I was owed for doing the sessions that are highlighted in red here... to be paid at AAS rates....

'Now, I've spent the last sixteen years as a consultant, I've given my career's life's blood to fighting this kind of thing…[financial sharp practice] and to be accused of it myself, again, is just surreal, I just… (big sigh) couldn't handle it and something in me snapped when I finally got round to reading the detail of this at the weekend and went through particularly the stuff on the last but one page where there's even a threat here to go back through the previous paper submissions and extract money from me, recoup is I think the word here…. Ah, let's be quite clear here, for the record, there are claims here that about half of the sessions I've done are part-sessions and I've claimed for full ones, about a quarter of them I haven't done and about another quarter of them I have claimed when I'm already paid to be doing something in the Trust?

'OK, let's just be clear, this is false. OK? This is false. Utterly false. And it's outrageous that I've been accused of this. OK? And it would have taken… 90 seconds… to have given Pamela Athersmith a call? Pam knows what were up to in the department. Pam could have told you this is false. Yeah? It was false. And that's what triggered my resignation. I just thought "I get the message", and I've got the message….'

Already aware of the other protests from within the Critical Care Division, it is no surprise that my very emphatic and heartfelt objections went uncontested by anyone in the room.

We moved on to some of the contemporary issues with safety in the department. I continued,

'And there was another case, you know, if anything's more serious than an infected obstructed kidney then it's an infected obstructed single kidney. We had another….'

Amidst expressions of disbelief I went on….

'Again, again. So, patient pitched up at FGH, not just septic but in renal failure as well with a hydronephrotic [blocked] single kidney late afternoon, can't remember what day of the week. Consultant on-call at Lancaster said "admit to ICU and haemo-filter." OK? That's a bit like having a tension pneumothorax and saying admit to ICU and ventilate. OK? You're not addressing the problem. OK? Patient should have been stented. OK? I picked up the case by accident next morning when I was seeing someone else. There wasn't even a plan of theatre then. The patient was sitting up in bed having their breakfast so they weren't even starved ([fasted: a pre-requisite for surgery]. (Sigh) So I rushed them off to theatre that afternoon and again I didn't bother putting in a clinical incident form because...? What's the point? So I'm afraid.... So the department is **not** safe....

So, even setting aside all this money I'm owed, I don't belong in this department any-more. I **cannot** work with clinical standards that are this low, that are this dangerous and where we seem to be just incapable of dealing with it.'

Becoming quite emotional, I went on to state...

'This has been going on for...12, 18 months, we've had near miss after near miss.... We've had the coroner's case, the [Patient A case], avoidable death, you know, **we do not learn** as a department, **we do not learn**, and, like I said, I've just come to the end of my tether with it all...'

The meeting moved on to behavioural issues in the department, provoking another impassioned intervention from myself.

'OK, so **what** have I been accused of, other than whistle-blowing and trying to keep standards high in the department? **What** have I actually been accused of? What substantially inappropriate behaviour, other than trying to oppose things like fraudulent behaviour ... and so on, what have I actually been accused of?'

It was towards the end of the meeting that the truly shattering revelation was finally dragged out of the senior managers and clinicians. I had been the subject of a triple racism allegation. Had I not doggedly persisted with my questioning of Dr Walker and Ms Joshi, I'm in no doubt that this crucial fact would never have emerged. This joint allegation was reluctantly described as being historic, perhaps 18 months earlier and I guessed at the time (correctly) that it had happened in the run up to my having to leave RLI and was perhaps the trigger for the NHS involving the clinical psychologists. The meeting was told that Mr Madhra, Mr Jain and Mr Naseem had all been *extremely outspoken* about my racism. It was also conceded that these allegations had been made in front of a senior NHS manager and the minutes subsequently circulated within the Trust.

Informed that the allegations had all been very non-specific and that the Trust had been unable to act against me as a consequence, it brought a heartfelt response from myself. The bare text entirely fails to convey the emotion.

'There won't be any specifics! Because I'm <u>not</u> a racist! It's <u>that</u> easy!'

'No….' was the answer.

I finally saw the minutes of that fateful meeting of late 2014, where I'd first been labelled a racist, some 18 months later in March 2018, over three years after they'd been made. At that point, just a few weeks before my Employment Tribunal hearing I learned for the very first time that the meeting was also attended by an external observer from the British Association of Physicians of Indian Origin/Medical Defence Shield adviser.

It is impossible to put into words how big a shock this revelation was to me, coming just days after I'd been forced into unemployment. It also came less than a year after I had been explicitly reassured that nothing like this had happened during my meeting with Dr Walker in late 2015 and had been made to look rather silly and paranoid when I had again expressed my fears of a two-way racism allegation in my meeting with Dr Walker and Ms Joshi in 2016. I had another distinct 'out of body' moment and, coming on top of my forced resignation and the sheer lunacy of the fact that I was now simultaneously the Trust's Doctor of the Year yet also illegally sacked and forcibly unemployed, the whole situation seemed utterly utterly absurd, surreal and disorientating.

The atmosphere of the meeting changed at this point and I was tentatively offered the chance to withdraw my resignation. I said that I would think about it. I was desperate to get out of there without being sick, get some fresh air and get my head around this truly career-ending bombshell.

After a rather rambling and semi-incoherent conversation with Colin Cutting in the car-park, I tried to drive back to the RLI. However, perhaps half a mile after leaving the hospital I was finally overcome with the enormity of it all and pulled over into a lay-by on the way out of Kendal, sitting trembling and shaking with my head in my hands for some half an hour, feeling the thuds from the ventricular ectopics rolling across my chest and praying that my heart would start up again after each compensatory pause. Finally, I felt composed and safe enough to start the car up again and drive home and tell Fiona what had happened. We agreed that with three historic and uncontested racism allegations against my name that had been festering for years and would appear to have been circulated around the organisation and outside it to BAPIO, together with perhaps even more damaging and equally, utterly false accusations amounting to attempted fraud from the Critical Care Division, unless UHMB came up with something truly exceptional, my career in the NHS and possibly even my registration as a doctor was over, once and for all and for ever.

I DON'T REMEMBER MUCH of the few days and weeks that followed. I was dazed and bewildered that in the space of a few months I had gone from joint departmental lead and Morecambe Bay's Doctor of the Year, to being forced into resignation, unemployed and possibly unemployable, with uncontested allegations of racism and attempted fraud against my name, allegations that numerous individuals within the Trust itself knew full well to be false. My sense of disbelief was heightened further still by a phone call from an old colleague, revealing that the resignation of my old and much loved senior colleague, Dick Wilson had also been precipitated by a similar campaign waged against him.

I was asked back urgently to a further meeting with Dr Walker and Ms Joshi a week or so later. I hadn't got the minutes from the first meeting at that point and therefore asked that these be provided before I agreed. I was also rather hesitant as Ms Joshi had been very short and abrasive with me and it was noticeable that neither Mr Cutting nor Ms Pharoah had been invited to the second meeting. As I felt that I could at least rely on these two individuals, their being left out troubled me significantly. I noted in an email to Jodie Brownlie of the Trust's HR department that I had found the initial meeting very stressful and traumatic.

The minutes were finally provided and I then agreed to a further meeting, waiting for a date to be fixed. Colin and Belinda were also still pushing to see if I could be re-employed and I continued to make clear my availability for further meetings in the hope-against-hope that UHMB could somehow come up with some kind of package that might enable me to resume work for the NHS with some modicum of safety.

I was subsequently rather rudely told by Morecambe Bay's HR Department on 7th December that as I had initiated an Employment Tribunal claim, Morecambe Bay would have no further meetings with me.

With regard to your request for a second meeting – As you are no longer employed by the Trust and pursuing a claim via an Employment Tribunal, it would not be appropriate to arrange further meetings.

I had deliberately left submitting a legal claim to the very last minute in the hope of some kind of sensible resolution or negotiated settlement. Even at this stage, it seemed incredible that I might end up taking legal action against the very Trust that I'd given my best sixteen years of service to and the organisation (the NHS) that I'd committed my adult life to serving. However, I had to place my claim, otherwise it would have become time expired.

There is a strict three month time limit to Employment Tribunal claims. As I've become more worldly-wise in the issues of employment law, I've increasingly suspected that this was part of the NHS's tactic, to try to draw the process out until I would have no claim in law and the whole issue was time-expired.

In one of my final conversations with the Care Quality Commission in late 2016 I was told that UHMB had assured the CQC that it was doing everything possible to re-recruit me. My contact at the CQC was clearly shocked when I read out the email telling me that there would be no more meetings and was equally shocked to hear that UHMB had already advertised, interviewed and recruited my successor and hence there was no job for me to come back to anyway.

It is worth pointing out that recruiting a new consultant normally takes many, many months of negotiation and discussion, with numerous committees in the NHS having to authorise the job, even before a formal advertisement is put out. I was astonished therefore to see that the advert for my successor had been rushed through so quickly. It was apparent that the two PDF documents advertising my post and detailing the job and person specification were created on 13th September 2016, way before I had worked out my notice and well before we even had the first meeting date arranged.

Looking back at the foot-dragging and delays that went on in association with my one and only meeting with any of the Trust's executives, the refusal to meet until I'd worked out my notice and was unemployed, the refusal to meet again and the breakneck speed with which the Trust recruited my successor, I clearly and belatedly drew the unavoidable conclusion.

UHMB were clearly determined that there was to be no way back into the organisation for me and had never the slightest intention of allowing any possibility of compromise.

There were no further meetings.

PART II

Litigation and the Isle of Man

CHAPTER ONE

Unemployment and a new job

LATE 2016 WAS a truly terrible period for both me and for the extended family. Unemployed and suddenly missing the monthly income from my NHS job, it was terrifying how fast the family finances went into reverse. Bills, of course, keep coming in and after nearly 30 years of regular work and earning a solid, steady income, it was deeply disturbing to suddenly find myself out of a job whilst our current account rapidly disappeared deep underwater.

I emailed a number of locum agencies during this period to see if I could get temporary work, explaining my circumstances and difficulties with Morecambe Bay and enclosing a copy of my CV. None replied, perhaps mindful of offending a powerful regional employer of locum staff, or perhaps because I'd already been black-listed. Having been warned by colleagues and managers that BAPIO and the local BME (Black and Minority Ethnic) group had been involved in my case, I'd already mentally written off any prospect of a regular job within the region. I felt that it would have left me too vulnerable to further retribution, particularly as several of my ex-colleagues held honorary or part time posts elsewhere around the region. Had I taken up a post within commuting distance of Lancaster, it seemed only a short matter of time until the false allegations caught up with me and the witch-hunt resumed.

It is difficult to articulate how awful those weeks were. Ever since my late teens, I'd worked single-mindedly towards getting a consultant surgeon's post in the Morecambe Bay area. Having had that achievement torn away from me, I was left with a sense of complete disorientation. Wandering around the house in a daze, I'd find myself falling asleep at inappropriate hours, dreaming of my old job, or having nightmares about the demotion, pay cut or the meeting where the extent of the witch-hunt against me had been revealed. Nights seemed never ending with sleep in short supply and nightmares my constant companion.

I don't recall much of that period other than the overwhelming and contradictory feeling of both anxiety and lethargy and of being dazed by the speed and brutality with which I'd been dismissed, whilst still holding the Trust's 'Doctor of the Year' award. I was aware that Colin, Belinda and other colleagues were loyally continuing to point out the completely fictitious nature of the allegations against me and were lobbying hard for another meeting between myself and the Trust. I think that by this point, however, they too were exhausted, dispirited and seemed to be getting nowhere with such requests.

Approached by ex-colleagues abroad who had heard of my predicament, I was by December 2016 at the point of seriously discussing posts in either the Middle East or even New Zealand. Fiona and I had cashed in £45,000 of our retirement savings to keep the family afloat and try and get our current account back into the black. I was getting really desperate when, mid-morning one weekday, I took a call from Chris Till.

Chris was an old friend, colleague and consultant anaesthetist from Morecambe Bay. I'd rather lost touch with him after my move to Furness General, but it turned out that he'd moved on to pastures new, working for Noble's Hospital on the Isle of Man, preceded there by another anaesthetic colleague from Lancaster, Dave Highley.

Chris's call was short and to the point. They had a long term locum urology middle grade position on the Isle of Man. Would I be interested in taking this up, except at regular rather than locum rates?

Rather like the arrangement that took me to Furness General, this made perfect sense. It would cost Noble's a lot less than an agency locum middle grade and would supply the island with a second consultant. Chris did a good recruiting job, painting a picture of a considerably healthier working environment than I'd been used to.

In my desperate position the offer seemed like a rope thrown to a drowning man.

A week later and I'd booked a day return ticket on the Isle of Man ferry from Heysham. This is not (with the benefit of hindsight) something that I'd recommend. Departing from Heysham Port at 2.15am, I stepped onto Manx soil for the first time at 6am, bleary and baggy eyed, unshaven, befuddled and slightly seasick. The return journey began at 7.45pm and I staggered back off the boat at 11.30pm the same evening, back where I'd started, seasick again, sleep deprived, desperately in need of a shower and more disorientated than ever.

However, the trip changed everything. Noble's Hospital was bright, clean, cheery and pleasant and whilst it seemed clear that the Manx health service was not awash with money, the impression was a world away from the overstretched service that I'd left. The nursing staff were particularly impressive, with the wards appearing cheerful, efficient, well-staffed and well run. I was left with the overwhelming impression of a healthy and functioning service, without the overstretched, dangerous feeling of the NHS, nor the obsession with hitting artificial and often unhelpful targets. Introduced to Steve Upsdell (the incumbent consultant urological surgeon), Jackie and Marie (the Urology specialist nurses) and Julie, (the urology secretary, but in reality more like a super-efficient PA), I was deeply impressed with the efficiency and functionality of the department.

By the following day I'd already contacted Oliver, the surgical manager at Noble's and in what seemed like record time, I'd been offered a job 'on the bank', being paid at an hourly rate whilst a longer term post was sorted out.

LEAVING THE FAMILY and family home, friends and relatives for a new job overseas was deeply disorientating and a definitive new lifetime low.

I booked my second crossing from Birkenhead on Sunday 18th December on the Isle of Man Steam-Packet ferry, the Ben-My-Chree, otherwise known simply as 'The Ben' to those on the island. Packing the boot of my ageing 3 series BMW with essential clothing and a few other meagre personal items and food supplies was profoundly depressing. Looking back at our lovely house with all its family memories of the boys growing up, I wondered how long it would be until I could properly regard it as home again. However, my mood then was as nothing compared with my emotions as the Ben slipped away down a grey and dismal-looking Mersey on the Sunday afternoon. Raining heavily out of an equally grey and sullen sky, I shared the freezing outside deck with a small handful of sodden and shivering, die-hard smokers. Still, as the last sights of England faded into the rain and murk, I comforted myself with the fact that the rain trickling down my cheeks at least meant that none of my companions could see that, for the first time since my teens, I was crying.

CHAPTER TWO

Litigation

LATE 2016 WAS, in addition to my increasingly desperate search for work, the time when the likelihood of litigation first seriously presented itself. I'd been in touch with the BMA for some considerable time, initially about my pay-cut and then about the demotion and the threat to move my base hospital. The utterly brutal events of summer 2016 clearly made my resignation inevitable. Having initially encouraged me to try and ride things out, by July the BMA themselves agreed that I'd been given no choice but to protect myself from further retaliation by handing my notice in, especially with the refusal of Morecambe Bay to honour payment for £36,000 of work that I'd done and the 'sting-in-the-tail' threat to go back through my prior earnings, recouping monies.

There seemed no prospect of any assistance from the CQC at this point. Although I'd continued to speak to my contact there on a regular basis (and it seemed clear that she was very shocked at the speed and ferocity of the backlash against me), it was made equally clear that, much to my dismay, the CQC would not intervene on my behalf. Similarly, although the CQC inspected Morecambe Bay in late 2016, my contacts in the department reported that the inspectors seemed to have gone out of their way to avoid the urology department. Not a single member of staff from urology was spoken to and no questions were asked about the avoidable death and disobedience to the Coroner. This was despite my having provided the CQC with a list of names and contact numbers of about 8-12 people to talk to (including, for fairness, those individuals who had made the allegations about me).

There was much speculation that the CQC didn't want to find anything that might involve them having to reverse their decision to take the Morecambe Bay NHS Trust out of special measures.

As 2016 morphed into 2017, I wrote with increasing desperation to NHS Improvement, NHS England, the National Guardians Office, (part of the CQC, responsible for NHS whistle-blowers), Jeremy Hunt's office at the Department of Health and even the Parliamentary sub-committee for Health and the Equality and Human Rights Commission. Each and every one dismissed my desperate pleas for help and support with the exception of the Parliamentary committee, who simply didn't bother to reply.

The prize for the most obtuse reply undoubtedly goes to the Equality and Human Rights Commission, whose response left me in frank disbelief. It claimed that whilst I might feel that I'd suffered extreme prejudice, hatred and discrimination as a consequence of my strong beliefs in safe care for NHS patients, the Equality Act didn't apply to me as I didn't have a protected characteristic.

How on earth, I mused in disbelief, can it then be called the Equality Act when the act itself discriminates on the basis of personal characteristics?

My local MP, Cat Smith was helpful and understanding but felt, I think, a little powerless to help. Litigation seemed the only way left in which I might get some kind of justice or vindication. Little did I appreciate just how savage and corrupt the process would be.

CHAPTER THREE

Getting the case together

BY LATE AUTUMN OF 2016 it was clear that, as far as Morecambe Bay and the NHS was concerned, I was dead and buried career-wise. The three month deadline for submitting a legal Employment Tribunal claim had come and gone and I'd been forced to put in a claim to avoid it being time-expired. Seemingly desperate to fill my post in record time, Morecambe Bay had already put out an advert for my job and shortlisted candidates. Frustrated, perhaps by the fact that I'd got in my legal claim just within the time limits, the Trust responded by making it clear that I was utterly out in the cold.

Thankfully I'd been a member of the British Medical Association for many years and, having always rather grudgingly paid the subscriptions, my membership now proved to be invaluable. The BMA had been well aware of my difficulties and anxieties regarding the Trust and clinical standards, going back several years. Although they'd previously been against my resignation, having seen the Job Plan Review document and accepting that senior management clearly had no intention of reversing the accusations contained within it they now agreed that the NHS had given me no choice over my resignation. At their request I prepared a summary of my position for assessment of whether they would support me in taking legal action.

The BMA's threshold for legal action is whether the case has a better than 50:50 chance of winning in any subsequent litigation. Having cleared this hurdle, my case was passed on to Gateley's Solicitors and Chris Thompson. Chris also applied the same criteria to my case and made the same judgement. The BMA do not them-selves litigate and therefore use Gateley's as an independent source of advice and litigation on their behalf. Chris was to become a regular and valued confidante and adviser to me over the next two years.

It is worth pointing out at this juncture that to have taken the case to an Employment Tribunal myself and with self-funded legal help would have been ruinously expensive and it is not at all uncommon for litigants to run up bills of six figures. The alternative, fighting the case myself and without expert legal help would undoubtedly have meant me falling at the first hurdle, such are the complexities of the Employment Tribunal process. Thankfully, my costs were covered but, although the BMA will pick up personal legal costs, they will not cover a costs award against a claimant, as I was to be painfully reminded of later in the process.

Chris helped me to put together our initial case and this was submitted within the three month limit for such claims. For anyone contemplating this kind of action it is worth noting that the Employment Tribunals are very inflexible over this. Miss the three month deadline and, unless you have an exceptionally good reason, your case is as good as lost.

My case evolved over several discussions with Chris and ultimately became a case for unfair constructive dismissal (essentially unfair sacking) and detriments (punishments) as a consequence of the Trust's behaviour. I strongly believed (as did absolutely everyone else in the department) that the only credible reason for my punishments and dismissal was the fact that I'd proved to be a threat to the Trust and its management by making protected disclosures (blowing the whistle) on serious safety related issues, most notably the avoidable death and disobedience to HM Coroner, over which I had of course gone to the CQC.

Linking the whistle-blowing to the constructive dismissal claim brought my case under the powers of the Public Interest Disclosure Act (PIDA). Drawn up by Parliament in 1999, it was designed to offer unlimited compensation to whistle-blowers who suffer detriment or dismissal as a result of their protected disclosures or whistle-blowing. However, as I was to come to learn the hard way, there are ways and means of circumventing the good intentions of this legislation. Large NHS Trusts, their HR Departments and their teams of lawyers are of course frequent flyers and experts at playing the system in such cases.

Litigation against a large and powerful £100 billion monopoly employer and public sector organisation like the NHS is a truly terrifying experience. Nothing in life prepared me for just what a bruising experience this would prove to be. Morecambe Bay responded almost immediately to our initial legal pleadings by trying to register a counter-claim against me, claiming that I had been invoicing for work that I hadn't done; again, essentially accusing me of fraud despite the fact that such claims had already been entirely discredited from within the Trust itself. *Details of the specific amounts... will be provided in due course.*

Thankfully, Chris quickly dealt with this but, aware as I was that the claims were not only entirely fictitious, but it was actually the Trust who had defrauded me, it was a first taste of kind of ruthless legal tactics that would be deployed against me over the next 18 months.

We can, of course, only speculate as to what might have happened to me next had Chris failed to get UHMB's counter claim struck out and had the Trust indeed been given a free hand to put together a case against me for NHS fraud.

Despite the terrible fear, danger and stress of all of this, in the midst of all of the claims and counter-claims was a moment of high farce and gross hypocrisy that had me emitting my biggest belly-laugh in years. UHMB's formal legal response to the Tribunal and reply to our original case contained an indignant, belligerent and seemingly heartfelt blanket denial of any illegal salary deduction or any other action on their part that might have constituted constructive dismissal.

> *The Claimant has been paid in accordance with his contract of employment and agreed Job Plan and it is denied that the Respondent made an unlawful deduction from the claimants wages as alleged or at all.*

The response also contained a restatement of the fiction that I'd been caught out over-invoicing.

Completely contradicting their judicial position, someone from the Trust had carefully and accidentally entered in the margins of the same legal letter a detailed summary of some of the sums of money that Morecambe Bay had deducted from my earnings.

It was a primary-school-level howler and moment of sublime comedy, bringing Fiona and the boys rushing into the room to see what had triggered the sudden roar of laughter followed by choking and snorting noises as I tried to get my breath back. Sadly, Chris, after enjoying a good laugh himself, told me that this might not be admissible as evidence of Morecambe Bay's dishonest and malign intentions towards me and the Employment Tribunal. Sure enough, it was ruled as being in-admissible in a subsequent preliminary hearing.

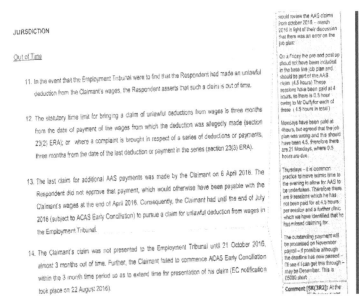

CHAPTER FOUR

Evidence, delays and preliminary hearings

BY LATE 2016 and extending all the way forward to 2018, my main priority was to try and get as much supportive evidence as I could. To describe this process as frustrating would be a major understatement.

Evidence to an Employment Tribunal can be roughly subdivided into written evidence (nowadays mostly emails, but also internal reports, minutes of meetings etc.) and witness statements from eyewitnesses who are prepared to give evidence in the Tribunal. As I was to painfully learn, the employer (or Respondent, as they are known in legal terms) has a monopoly on all of these.

From late 2016 on, a number of emails requesting evidence were exchanged between myself, Jodie Brownlie and then Claire Largue of the UHMB Human Resources Department. These centred around my request for information about what had happened using a subject access request (which we are all legally allowed to make under the Data Protection Act). I and the rest of the department were absolutely convinced that I'd been constructively dismissed as a consequence of going outside the organisation to the CQC, particularly over the highly toxic issues of the avoidable death and disobedience to HM Coroner.

It seemed logical to look for hard evidence of this in the emails that had been circulated about me amongst senior staff, colleagues and the members of the Board in the run-up to and after my resignation. However, it was clear very early on that the Trust was being as obstructive as possible, despite the requirement that each side provide all the evidence in their possession whether it supports their case or not.

Subject access requests made under the Data Protection Act are supposed to be dealt with within a month at the most. After hugely breaching the deadline for a response, I was finally informed that the NHS had located 11,000 emails. After a further huge delay, a tiny proportion of around 200 emails were finally and very grudgingly divulged sometime in 2017. Each and every one of them was redacted beyond any readability. A small number are reproduced here.

University Hospitals **NHS**
of Morecambe Bay
NHS Foundation Trust

Incident Details With Feedback

	PSI		SUI				

Subjects Of Incident	ID1	D.O.B	Staff/Person/Other	Role
Peter Duffy		/ /	(Other)	

Incident Details

Incident Description

Quality & Governance Team Comments

27/01/2017

183

PETER DUFFY

University Hospitals **NHS**
of Morecambe Bay
NHS Foundation Trust

Incident Details With Feedback

Investigation Details

27/01/2017

184

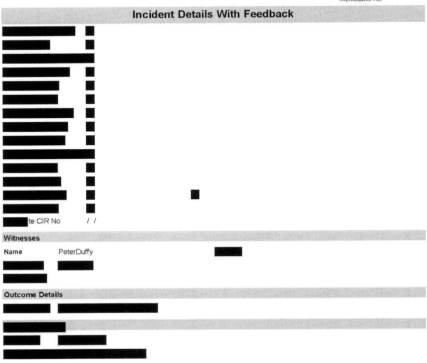

Incident Details With Feedback

University Hospitals **NHS**
of Morecambe Bay
NHS Foundation Trust

te CIR No   / /

Witnesses

Name   PeterDuffy

Outcome Details

Meanwhile, I was also told by Chris that I needed to start getting witnesses together, and that I should concentrate on securing the testimony of individuals from the department who had personal insights into what had happened and who would be able to put my punishments and dismissal into the appropriate context of overt whistle-blower retaliation.

Triumphantly, I read out to him the names of roughly ten people who had provisionally agreed to be witnesses for me and to support my version of events. Chris's response was dour and downbeat, 'You'll be lucky if even 10% of your witnesses go through with this.' He was to be proved, as usual, quite right.

Looking back, I was incredibly naive about the litigation process. I can imagine how difficult it must be for an experienced employment solicitor like Chris to have a series of clients come before you, each convinced that they have a completely unlosable, watertight case and that the process will be conducted in an atmosphere of politeness and mutual respect. It must be like watching a procession of innocent lambs being led to a particularly nasty slaughtering. To his credit, Chris did his best to play down my expectations, telling me to expect the NHS to approach the litigation process with all the fairness, tact and subtlety of a wild-west shoot-out. Again, he was spot-on.

In the background and away from the legal issues there was an exchange of emails with Mr Pearse Butler, UHMB chair in late 2016 to early 2017 and an offer was made to arrange meetings with the relevant people. This, of course, never happened. With the ongoing refusal of the Trust to provide any kind of meaningful disclosure following my Data Protection Act requests, it was at this point that I gave up any hope of resolving the issues informally.

In late January 2017 I was asked out of the blue by Dr Walker, Medical Director of UHMB, to supply a list of the more important clinical issues and incidents that I had flagged up. I prepared a detailed document of 27 cases that I had been involved in and reported (still only a small proportion of all the clinical issues over the previous years) and submitted this back.

In response and after a delay of some months, the Trust produced a document entitled 'SUMMARY REVIEW AND FINDINGS FOR PD: UROLOGY INCIDENTS'. This, however, only documented the investigation of some eight selected cases and even these investigations were in my opinion superficial, inadequate or downright misleading. In one case a young man who had been left impotent was categorised as a 'near miss'! This did not stop the Trust subsequently writing to NHS Improvement (NHSI), assuring them that I had suffered no detriment and that all the incidents that I had raised had been satisfactorily investigated.

In fact, it appears that only eight of the 27 cases have ever received any attention at all.

At roughly the same time and in addition to the assurances made to NHSI, the Trust told the CQC that the Tribunal hearing was simply to do with money issues:

> *Essentially, the Tribunal Hearing was initially about money and a Job Plan Review. There had been an informal agreement that the former member of staff could claim for additional activities. However, upon investigation it was identified that the member of staff was not always present on the dates when claims were made. This element of the claim has now been withdrawn. UHMB has paid the legitimate element of the claim.*

Not only was this completely and utterly untrue, but UHMB were all too well aware that it was untrue. Nevertheless, it seemed to convince the CQC that there was a problem with my probity, honesty and trustworthiness. It is perhaps no coincidence that the CQC showed no further interest in my case from this point on.

CHAPTER FIVE

Costs threats and a potential £108,000 bill

MUCH OF 2017 seemed to be spent in waiting. I busied myself with settling into my new job at Noble's Hospital, moving out of the cramped, shared hospital accommodation into the rented, under-the-eaves rooftop flat that I still occupy in Peel, a small and quaint town and fishing port on the west coast of the Isle of Man, not unlike Cornwall some 50 years ago. The Manx locals call this stretch of coast 'The Wild West' on account of the westerly winds and storms that crash in off the Irish Sea at regular intervals over the winter. Peel seafront at high tide and in a strong north-westerly can be a spectacular if not downright frightening place.

In July I was formally interviewed and appointed to a permanent position at Noble's Hospital and enjoyed a round of hugs, kisses, handshakes, high-fives and back-slapping from staff at all levels. They seemed genuinely delighted at my appointment and, although I was still separated from family and friends for the foreseeable future, at least we all now had once again the security of a regular income to supplement Fiona's part time GP earnings.

At last, I could start to think about the future and for the next year, this meant the run-in to the Tribunal case.

At the moment the wait for an employment law case like mine seems to be about 18 months. My own case was drawn out longer due to some of the preliminary hearings. It was at one of these in late 2016 that I first came across the impressive Judge Franey who would preside over the definitive hearings.

In summer of 2017 I took a call from Dr David Walker regarding the ongoing issues in the urology department. Ranging over a number of issues, we touched on the issue of the racism allegations made against me. Discussing the power and toxicity that such allegations carry and the intervention of BAPIO (the British Association of Physicians of Indian Origin) in the case, I made my fears clear,

'Um, there's no way I can possibly come back under those kind of circumstances because they'll... they'll nail me again. Erm, we know there's this racism allegation that is in writing, that's been circulating for quite a while which obviously I was completely unaware of.

'I mean, for me that doesn't just make it impossible for me to come back to Morecambe Bay, it makes it impossible for me to come back to NHS North West. You know, the sheer hatred that went into that and the toxicity of such a, an allegation, even though we all know that it's utterly false and it's utterly malicious and it's purely revenge for the clinical incidents that I've flagged up.

'Ah, so to have a three-way tactical racism allegation against me... ah, to me it really is akin almost to a kind of hate crime. You know, it'd have been better if they'd waited for me with baseball bats outside the hospital entrance because at least you can get better from that... ah...'

I was told in response that 'National BAPIO' had made the similar allegations about at least one other within the Trust.

My response was emphatic:

'Dear God...! I mean, with all due respect..., should this not be going right up to the top of the NHS? There's no way people... should be being held hostage...'

We went on to discuss a previous avoidable death (different from Patient A) that had happened in around 2010-11 at FGH.

'Yeah, bear in mind at the time I was very much trying to keep the peace with Kavinder (Madhra) back in place and just try and clear up the mess behind people without trying to attract more... anger.

'You could sense the department was starting the slippery slide again, but for a long time I held off any kind of direct criticism or reflection on other peoples' practice because I didn't want to end up in precisely in the kind of situation that of course I'm in.

'It was an appalling situation. I do remember first walking in. Again, it's one of the cases I still get nightmares about. Poor woman, just lying there semi-conscious in her own pus, discharging through her groin and all I could see that had been done was different antibiotics tried.... So as soon as I walked through that door I thought... *I'm too late here...* and she was cachectic and you just think... *ohhh* <u>*s**t*</u>, you know, *I'm going to lose this woman whatever I do....* So that was bad, yeah....'

We went on to discuss the two single-kidney cases from 2014 that had been left without stents.

'To be honest with you as well, part of the reason I phoned them was because by this stage I had put in so many incidents, you know, I'd gone through the point of raising things informally. I'd gone through the point of passing things on to ... who, I think was passing them on in turn. We got to the clinical incident stage and things weren't happening....

'And I thought if I just put an incident in about this, what'll happen is Ash (Jain)'ll be interviewed; he'll insist that the two colluded and it'll just be like, case closed, move on, next case. I thought I'm going to present.... I'm going to go and get my facts right, 'cos I knew he was telling lies and then I thought I will then pass it on to the division in such a way that they **have** to act. And so that was my motivation 'cos I was just sick of incident after incident that I felt was being covered up and of all those RCAs [root cause analyses] that you passed back to me I've only ever seen one. I was kept totally in the dark about the rest... I'd no idea.'

We went on to discuss the case of the avoidable death at Lancaster Royal Infirmary and the issues over the Coroner's orders; David

Walker pointing out to me the importance of obeying the Coroner's orders.

I replied:

'Oh, there's no doubt we disobeyed the Coroner over the [Patient A] case. Er, I even took the notes… A's notes, along to the morbidity and mortality meeting. Ash and Saleem said to me *We are not discussing that case.* His notes were in a great big bundle in a shopping bag so they were instantly recognisable and as soon as I walked in with them under my arm I was told, *No, we are not discussing that.*'

Told that I should have escalated that, I replied….

'Oh it was. Trust me. I certainly emailed… and possibly other people and I even drew the comparison with the Joshua Titcombe case saying, you know, as a Trust we cannot possibly afford, once again, to be trying to mislead the Coroner and play around with the Coroner's inquests and so on…. But it seemed to fall on deaf ears…'

Going on to discuss regulatory issues, I put my position on taking my concerns externally.

'No, well…. I guess, I've always been very nervous about going outside the Trust, er, because… we all tend to know what often happens to people who blow the whistle, and I do think that if I could be flagged up for making any mistakes during this, it's actually not going to the GMC and the CQC earlier, er…. It was just a bad call of mine. I was just too intimidated and I think also I was too…. Er…. I had quite a, a pretty awful time with my own GMC enquiry back in 2011 or whenever it was and I didn't really want to see them and their families put through something similar. But that was a bad call of mine… if I put my hand up to anything… any big mistakes it's that. I really should have gone… to the GMC many years ago…. But there we are, I kind of trusted people internally to sort it out….'

Finishing up, I returned to my disbelief over some of the revelations earlier in the conversation.

'I do think, just to re-iterate what I said, erm, if this is as wide-spread as I think it is across the NHS it is incredibly toxic. You know, if you've got good clinicians... and good managers being threatened with racism allegations if they're not doing what particular power groups want... you know, it starts to sound like a kind of mafia-type setup doesn't it, where you're getting people blackmailed and threatened and decisions skewed and corrupted....'

AFTER THAT, little of consequence happened in 2017, although as the year closed there was a distinct sense of things starting to speed up.

The run in to a Tribunal hearing is a bit like landing an aeroplane. From high up and a long way away, everything seems to happen slowly and gradually. But as the runway comes closer, things start to speed up and suddenly, in the last moments before landing, everything seems to be rushing past at a terrifying speed.

Frustrated by the Trust's refusal to provide the vital evidence that we needed, Chris took our case to a preliminary hearing in early 2018 to force the NHS to provide the evidence that we knew that it was continuing to with-hold. In this respect we were at least partially successful, one major concession being that I finally got to see, some four years after it was produced, the minutes of the meeting where I had been accused of being a racist by Mr Madhra, Mr Jain and Mr Naseem, together with the anonymised note to the Police, accusing me of being a racist and a bully. Incredibly and to my great anger and indignation, the minutes of the secret meeting revealed that, seemingly without any prior warning or discussion with the Trust, an observer from the British Association of Physicians of Indian Origin (BAPIO) had turned up to witness the whole thing. It seemed unbelievable that potent allegations, including what I was assured were *outspoken* (and almost certainly defamatory) allegations of racism against myself were made, not only without giving me any chance to respond, but without my even being aware of the briefings that were going on behind my back.

The written evidence started to pile up and it became a major job sorting through it all and sifting it into piles of the relevant and irrelevant.

It's an odd feeling, going through emails that feature you, but where the authors clearly never meant for you to be aware of their comments. Most of the information was irrelevant but there were some shocks, as well as recognition of how hard Colin Cutting had fought my corner. There were emails and grievances from Mr Jain and Mr Naseem that again clearly implied racism on my part and, astonishingly and shortly later, a slew of secretive emails from within the Critical Care Division, centred round an accusation that I was costing the division over £100,000 per year in non-productivity. Even more astonishingly, the figure was produced by a manager within the division whom I regarded as a friend, yet the emails clearly implied truly massive wastage and inefficiency, despite the validation efforts (of which he was fully aware) probably having saved that very same division a six-figure sum.

£112,340 was the annual sum of money in question. Each email was headlined as highly important and confidential and referred to what sounded like secretive divisional briefings and covert meetings about me.

It all sounded so ridiculously melodramatic that I almost laughed out loud, expecting a subheading of 'Top-secret! This message will self-destruct in 5 seconds!' accompanied by Mission Impossible music, stun grenades and Tom Cruise bursting through the door.

However, my amusement over such clearly false briefings faded when I reflected on the sheer amount of damage that these emails must have done to me. Once again, it appeared to me that false, fabricated and covert accusations had been doing the rounds, with no attempt made to stop them, counter them with the truth or allow me to answer or provide my side of the story.

Reflecting on the NHS's original threat to take legal counter-action against me, I was in no doubt that these allegations would have taken centre-stage in such proceedings. Shakily, I reflected on just how much it could have cost my family if Chris had failed to get the NHS's counter-claim struck out.

However, it was what was missing that was the most important and disappointing. No emails from Mr Madhra, no emails from Jackie Daniel (our chief executive), no significant emails to or from the other Trust Board members over my resignation, or from BAPIO or the regional BME group (who I had been assured had also put pressure on the Trust to act in favour of the colleagues that I had expressed concerns about). Despite the preliminary hearing, it seemed clear that we were not going to get full disclosure.

I was becoming increasingly frustrated over the lack of disclosure as the main hearing drew close but consoled myself with the thought that we still had the ace up our sleeve. Although there'd been a few drop-outs, I was confident that we could field six to eight witnesses from the department, all of whom were well aware of the chronology and would confirm what we all knew, namely that I had never taken money from the NHS illicitly; it was the other way round. I was entirely confident that they would support the overwhelming belief that I had been deliberately targeted for a fabricated contractual dispute. That I had been dismissed as a consequence of my taking my concerns over the Coroner's case to the CQC; and because of the pressure that my concerns and the counter-allegations had put on senior management over clinical and behavioural standards in the department.

And then disaster struck. The remaining consultants and middle grades were called together by the Trust sometime in perhaps early 2018, given a very severe dressing down and, according to several colleagues, informed that the Trust would seek to close or 'dissolve' the department if subsequent events went badly. It was, I was told, like being scolded by the headmaster.

At a stroke, all but one of my remaining witnesses dropped out. Some simply stopped replying to my emails or texts. Others quoted various other commitments or the *fear of God* being put into them whilst most simply quoted the old maxim about turkeys and voting for Christmas.

Chris had warned me about this and it seems to be a common tactic in these kinds of tribunals. Of course, with the NHS being a monopoly employer, its employees are particularly vulnerable to such manoeuvres and, having seen my own treatment at the hands of the NHS, I can't for one second blame my ex-colleagues for acting first and foremost to protect their own families and careers.

Colin Cutting was of course a vital witness and although I'd approached him some 18 months earlier, he had been informed right from the start of the litigation that he'd only be allowed to appear as a witness for the NHS. Having refused to sign the witness statement written out for him and insisted on writing his own account, he was subsequently informed that he'd not be allowed to appear at all, nor would his witness statement be seen by the Tribunal.

By the last fortnight before the Tribunal I had just one witness left. Alison Birtle, consultant clinical oncologist had been a close colleague and friend from about 2006. She, unlike my other witnesses had always been employed by a neighbouring Trust and was perhaps a little less affected and more detached. I struggle to think of anyone tougher or more articulate than Alison but even she seemed intimidated by the process and, as not strictly a member of the urology department, was unable to produce much detail on my treatment at the hands of my colleagues and management. Under such circumstances I was simply very, very grateful that someone had the courage to turn out and support me in the face of such hostility.

With a week to go to the Tribunal, I was a lot less certain of my prospects than I had been a year earlier. Witness statements had been exchanged and it seemed clear that the Trust's tactic would be to deny everything. If they were indeed found guilty of having illegally dismissed me, then they would fall back to a separate plea, claiming that it was an accident and a consequence of a contractual dispute triggered by inexperienced junior management. In one of the sworn statements, the allegation was again repeated that I had claimed £112,000 that I was potentially not entitled to.

Elsewhere was the allegation about me that *as far as we could tell, he was not even working the PAs* (half-day sessions) *that he was already being paid for...* The clear impression given by the Trust's witness statements was that my resignation was my fault for indulging in inappropriate false invoicing and that senior management had throughout the process been helpless and unable to intervene.

It was at this point that I began to fully realise just how much hatred I'd generated. The witch-hunt was still alive, well, thriving and pursuing me all the way into the Employment Tribunal.

I'd regarded the original £112,000 allegation against me as comically inept but here it was, being submitted to an Employment Tribunal under oath. I found it difficult to believe (and still do) that a colleague and fellow-professional would have made such a sworn statement, given that the facts were false and misrepresented. The Trust's team must have appreciated that if the false allegations were accepted by the Tribunal and hence given an additional veneer of authenticity, the implications of possible six-figure NHS fraud could pursue me all the way to a GMC hearing and even a criminal conviction, as well as losing me the case. It seemed that my ex-employer was prepared to level any kind of allegation against me, no matter how ridiculous and no matter what the potential consequences for me and my family, simply to try and justify my awful treatment at their hands.

These kinds of counter-allegations are a common tactic in litigation, known in legal circles as 'reason-shopping'. The Respondent (NHS) essentially denies everything, but also lays out a fall-back position where, if found guilty of constructive dismissal, it then claims that it was due to an aspect of the Claimant's history or behaviour unrelated to whistle-blowing.

There are two reasons for this.

Firstly, no Trust or large employer wants to be publicly caught out deliberately sacking or constructively dismissing a whistle-blower. Whilst an illegal sacking is bad publicity, it is a lot less damaging to be seen to have unfairly sacked someone for perceived financial irregularities or for personal differences than for doing their job and flagging up dangerous failings in the organisation. It's even better if the whistle-blower can be labelled as a possible fraudster and thus discredited, whilst any alleged management errors can be explained away as being the responsibility of junior managers, conveniently not called to give evidence and therefore unable to defend themselves.

The second reason for trying to provide an alternative explanation is cost. Tribunal compensation is capped by parliament and Tribunals are only allowed to award compensation to an upper limit. About £88,000 was the maximum sum for constructive dismissal in 2016. However, in constructive dismissal for whistle-blowing cases the cap is off and the damages are unlimited. Faced, as a consequence of the witch-hunt against me, with the prospect of having to live abroad and away from my family for another eight years and having already been separated from them for eighteen months, the costs could clearly climb quickly well into six figures. However, if the Trust could persuade the Tribunal that they'd dismissed me either accidentally or for reasons unrelated to my whistle-blowing then the £88,000 cap would be firmly screwed back on again.

I was well aware from an early stage that the Trust was reason-shopping my background and employment history very carefully indeed. I was told that at one point they had considered alighting on racism as a fall-back reason for my dismissal. Finding precisely no evidence to back this up and with these allegations completely contradicted by my 'Doctor of the Year' award, they'd then examined the ongoing and entirely fabricated issues over my probity and possible fraud. Finally, they seemed to have picked on 'accidental' dismissal as a consequence of the fake probity allegations as being the most credible alternative explanation to offer to the Tribunal in the event that they lost over the constructive dismissal claim.

Despite the withdrawal of so many witnesses and our failure to get full disclosure of the written evidence, I was still in a fairly robust and positive frame of mind in the last few days run-in to the Tribunal. I felt that I'd written a good, honest and balanced witness statement, exhaustingly cross-referenced to the bundle of what evidence had been declared and I still felt that our case was strong.

Then, with just four working days to go and after eighteen months of preparation, I received an urgent email from Chris. The Trust had sent a 'without prejudice save as to costs' letter. Could I get in touch ASAP?

A 'without prejudice' letter is a tactic that has its roots in a genuine attempt to facilitate out-of-court settlements. It allows a negotiating position to be laid out without the negotiator's position being legally compromised. For example, a penitent employer might make a financial offer of settlement to a wronged employee under such a heading. The 'without prejudice' aspect then prevents the letter from being revealed to the Tribunal and thus protects the employer from damaging or compromising their legal position by a written admission of weakness.

Unfortunately and as I have belatedly come to learn, such letters have moved well away from their original positive role and have in my opinion become weapons for further punishment, threats, intimidation and retaliation against whistle-blowers in Employment Tribunal cases.

Anyone preparing a similar case would be well advised to expect such a tactic and to prepare their response well ahead.

In my case, the letter was brutal in both its language and negotiating position. I was assured by the Trust's solicitors in the most intimidating language that I was doomed to lose every aspect of the case and that my pursuit of the case was unreasonable and vexatious. In the inevitable event of losing, I was assured that Morecambe Bay NHS Trust would then pursue me and my family for costs, estimated at £92,000 + VAT (£108,000).

If I agreed to drop my case immediately and in its entirety, stay silent and agree to a non-disclosure clause that was clearly intended to gag me then Morecambe Bay would not pursue costs.

The letter gave me two days to reply.

I DON'T RECALL MUCH from those last few days before the hearing began. I was absolutely numbed by the threat of the costs letter, particularly when it had been clear to all of us that one of Morecambe Bay's main defences was known by both sides to be false. Chris carefully explained that, whilst the BMA would pick up my own costs whatever the outcome, any award of the NHS's costs against me would have to be paid out of our family assets.

Of course, the only asset that we had that was worth six figures was the house. For several days, the family wrestled with what we should do.

None of us regarded this as anything other than full-on bullying, intimidation and blackmail.

Having based much of its case on a denial that the Trust knew to be false, having redacted emails and made comments that had precipitated the withdrawal of all my witnesses from Morecambe Bay itself, the Trust now seemed intent on threatening and intimidating me into withdrawing the case entirely. Chris, my solicitor and Paras Gorasia (who was to be my barrister and legal representative at the tribunal) were clearly of the opinion that this was no idle threat. The NHS, having already broken up the family and consigned me to living abroad for the rest of my career, was now perfectly prepared to try to wreck our family finances still further.

No words can adequately encompass my disbelief at this tactic. I still struggle to believe that something so intimidating is even legal, particularly where part of the threat was based on a denial that the Trust already knew to be false. I was equally disbelieving of the fact that it was seemingly acceptable to send such a document just four working days prior to the hearing, when the NHS had had eighteen months to prepare its defence. How did this tactic fit, I mused, with the NHS's promise, openly published on Morecambe Bay's 'Freedom to Speak Up' website, that no whistle-blower would lose their job or suffer any detriment?

Of course, there is no way of countering this kind of threat or intimidation. Even in the improbable event that a claimant like me was to make a counter threat of costs against the employer (Respondent), it would of course be pointless as in the case of the NHS, it would be the taxpayer who would pick up the tab, not the NHS managers and lawyers who were driving this abusive process.

After several sleepless nights, the family and I decided to proceed with the case, but also agreed that Paras, our barrister, would have a look at the case again over the weekend and would see if he could perhaps consolidate my case and my legal pleadings to try and minimise the risks of the NHS pursuing me for costs.

CHAPTER SIX

D Day

ON THE EVENING OF SUNDAY 15TH APRIL 2018, I carefully polished my best shoes, picked out my treasured Royal College of Surgeons tie and made sure that my favourite pinstripe suit still fitted me. Comfort eating is one of my weaknesses but luckily my extra ballast didn't seem to show too badly. I was determined to look my best, even after a string of sleepless nights and managed a joke with the family about trying to be the best-dressed lamb in the slaughter-house.

The train journey seemed interminable but at last I arrived at the Manchester Employment Tribunal. I'd arranged to meet Chris and Paras very early in order to go through our weekend thoughts and was again asked if I wanted to proceed, bearing in mind the ongoing threat of £108,000 costs.

I'd imagined that the Tribunal building would be a subdued, historic and dignified place, rather like a medieval library or cathedral, imbued with many years of legal history and quiet, intense learned argument. I couldn't have been more wrong. It was a huge concrete obscenity, there was an enormous queue waiting to go through security and, with about fourteen different Tribunal hearing rooms, the whole thing seemed to be organised on an industrial scale. I met up with Chris and Paras in the Claimants' room, again expecting it to be a quiet and secluded place. In fact, it was packed, the claimants easily picked out by their pale faces and pursed lips; their legal teams distinguished by the pinstripes, briefcases and easy detached confidence.

Paras had fleshed out a plan over the weekend and quickly explained it to me. We'd drop a fair number of my pleadings and would concentrate on one main protected disclosure (the Coroner's case) and two detriments; these being the failure to pay monies that were agreed, and the Job Plan Review document. These acts then formed the breaches that led to my resignation, constituting an act of unfair constructive dismissal. The association between the whistle-blowing and the detriment was the timing of the first pay cut, coming immediately after the CQC's opening of its investigation into the Trust's urology department in October.

Last-minute and hurried as it was, it seemed a good plan, leaving my substantive case in place whilst hopefully heading off, as best we could, the threat of costs.

Entering the court room for the first time is a pretty difficult thing to do. Of course, the Trust's team were there and I immediately recognised Gertie Nicphilib from Morecambe Bay's HR department as well as David Walker, the Medical Director. There was an awkward moment whilst I acknowledged these two individuals. Just a couple of years earlier I would have regarded them as close and trusted friends and colleagues. They were now part of a team that seemed determined to inflict even more damage on me and my family.

The Trust's team had already secured their places at the far side of the room, a good legal and psychological tactic that meant that I'd be completely separated from my own team when giving evidence, surrounded by the NHS's team on the one side, the Tribunal panel on the other and Paras on the far side of the room.

Having observed the formality of standing for the entrance of Judge Franey and the two other Tribunal members, Paras immediately got down to work, laying out my amended pleadings in legal language that I struggled to comprehend. With a sense of anti-climax, we were told that the Tribunal would take the rest of the Monday and the Tuesday to consider the revised pleadings and bundle (collection of written evidence) and would re-convene on Wednesday.

From the expressions and body language of the Trust's team, our refusal to buckle under the costs threat and the amended pleadings had not gone down at all well.

Regrouping on Wednesday, I was accompanied by Alison Birtle, consultant clinical oncologist based at Preston, my one remaining witness. Slightly farcically, the Trust's team had no questions for her about her witness statement and she was told, having got up especially early and travelled all the way down from Lancaster to Manchester, that she was free to go and travel all the way back!

Next up and much as I'd feared, I found myself taking the oath and my seat in the witness chair, with my back to the wall and surrounded very intimidatingly by the Trust's team and Tribunal panel. Morecambe Bay's barrister opened the questions for the NHS.

Being cross-examined under oath is a truly horrible experience and undoubtedly the most unpleasant experience of my life. Each question is carefully calculated to try and portray you in the worst possible light or alternatively to lead you away from the case that you are presenting and into a trap. Often there is a series of questions, each one deliberately couched to try and ensure a reply of 'yes' and each leading you towards the trap. All the time, a second lawyer for the NHS is frantically typing away to record every word that you utter. Notes are passed back and forth, with everything said being scrutinised and recorded, 'Ahh, Mr Duffy, can we take you back to something you said 45 minutes ago...?' Of course, by this time and under constant pressure, you can't quite remember exactly what it was that you said....

I think I managed to field each question fairly well until, just before lunch and when I was tired and probably at my most vulnerable, the trap was sprung.

I was asked a seemingly innocent question about the avoidable death case, the disobedience to the Coroner and my subsequent 'protected disclosure' in relation to this. Pressing me on precisely what constituted the protected disclosure, I told the Trust's barrister that it was my conversation to the CQC.

Wrong answer.

The Trust's lawyer gave a slow smile as I gave my reply. It was like a scalpel slash opening. 'That's not your pleaded case Mr Duffy,' he informed me with clear pleasure. There was a sudden sense of checkmate.

Paras intervened quickly to ask if the Tribunal would consider an amendment on my behalf. After listening to Paras's case, Judge Franey decided that it was time to break for lunch, suggesting that I discuss with Paras and Chris over lunch if I wished to pursue the case. The Tribunal would then consider whether such an amendment was reasonable. The judge warned me as I stepped down that I was still under oath and in purdah and, with the exception of speaking to Paras and Chris regarding my revised plea, I should not be party to any other influence that might affect my evidence giving. Astonishingly, despite this admonishment, I was quietly reminded from the Trust's team that I could still avert six-figure costs if I dropped the case and walked away.

Of course, lunch was the last thing on my mind and the overt and renewed threat left me completely sickened.

Sitting in the sunshine outside the Tribunal building, I spent perhaps an hour wrestling with the options. Calling Paras, jacking it all in and catching the first train home was an almost irresistible temptation and I could tangibly feel the draw of Salford Central station pulling me away from all of this and back to my family. *It would be so easy, to just pack it all in and walk away from the threat.* Of course, that was exactly what the Trust's legal team wanted. Feeling distinctly nauseated and with a heavy heart, I heaved myself upright and headed back to the Tribunal, with just a fleeting impression, as I glanced up, of someone in a hoodie, perhaps fifty metres away, smartly turning round a split second later, putting something down and walking away from me.

Did they just photograph me...?

Back in the building and with my heart throwing off ectopics right, left and centre, I told Paras and Chris that we'd continue and see if Judge Franey would allow the amended pleadings, fully aware that if I failed and my case collapsed, Morecambe Bay's NHS team would then pursue me for £108,000.

The Tribunal panel withdrew to consider the amended plea, re-convening after what seemed like an elephant's age (but was probably only five to ten minutes) to confirm to my huge relief that they would allow the amendment to go ahead. Within a few seconds and with hardly time to draw breath I was back in the witness box.

Luckily, I somehow managed to hold it all together that afternoon. However, there can be no doubt that the repeated costs threat had a major effect on my evidence. All afternoon, all I could think of was not annoying the Trust's legal team and Gertie Nicphilib in particular in case they did indeed decide to go through with their threat to come after me and my family for costs. Incredibly, at one point I was cross-examined about my medical history and attendances at Morecambe Bay's Occupational Health Department. Denying that I had ever knowingly missed an appointment and wondering what on earth this had to do with my case, it was clear that my answers were being transmitted back to Trust Headquarters and being scrutinised 'real-time' for any flaws in my evidence. Even my medical records didn't seem sacrosanct, with clearly audible and frantic tapping on Gertie's iPad at the back of the court room, the response being handed back minutes later on. Scribbled on a bit of paper was the rather shamefaced admission that I had indeed always attended any appointments. It all seemed positively Orwellian. Adam, another member of the team from Gateley's, commented the following day about how subdued and deferential to the Trust's legal team I had been throughout that afternoon.

Of course, I was warned again at the end of the day about speaking to third parties about anything that might affect my evidence and had to wait until after a sleepless night, lunch the following day and a further two to three hours of cross-examination before I was released from my oath and could speak to my legal team about how it was all going.

Paras and Adam felt that I'd done well under the circumstances, but were not very optimistic about proving the link between my resignation and whistle-blowing. The Trust's team, after steering me into the trap the previous day, had studiously avoided cross-examining me any further on this. Hence, with the withdrawal of all of my departmental colleagues from giving evidence and the redacting of emails, there was really very little hard evidence linking the two events for the Tribunal to reflect on.

Heading back into the Tribunal room for the afternoon session, I overheard the Trust's barrister whisper to Paras something about the case getting into the media. Paras threw a surprised look over his shoulder to the back of the Tribunal room. A young woman had been sitting there on the first day of the hearing and again during my cross-examination. I'd assumed she was with the Trust's team but now she was no longer there. I recalled the individual in the hoodie turning and walking away from me the previous day as I'd got up to go back into the Tribunal building.

Had I been covertly photographed? What on earth had the press said about me? Was I going to be accused of being a racist and an NHS fraudster in the national media too?

Thursday afternoon went in a blur. I tried to concentrate on what the Trust's witnesses were saying but was just too exhausted by the stress of it all. Relieved that the day was finally over, I staggered out, turning my mobile on only to find an email from 'Public Concern at Work'.

I was in the Daily Mail. Complete with photographs.

The article had clearly been culled from my witness statement with some sections repeated pretty much verbatim. I spent another sleepless night in turmoil, imaging the fury and hatred that was likely to be coming my way in the morning.

It is difficult to put into words just how terrified I was next morning. By now, the story was in several other national broadsheets and tabloids and, acutely aware of how hard the NHS had tried to close the case down and stop me from speaking out, I was so intimidated that I could barely force myself onto the train. My mental and physical state was so disturbed that I actually got off the train at one of the stations, shutting myself in the platform gents' toilets to check that I hadn't soiled myself.

Despite my impromptu pit-stop, I still arrived early at the Tribunal, whizzing in through the front door at supersonic speed to dodge any waiting press. No one seemed remotely interested in me and the Tribunal convened as normal.

The Trust's barrister was in like a flash. Had the Tribunal seen the media reports? The NHS had reason to believe that I had spoken to a journalist whilst under oath and thus broken purdah and compromised my evidence. The NHS requested that I be brought back for further cross-examination under oath about whether my case had been influenced by such illicit contact with a journalist.

Paras protested but Judge Franey announced that the Tribunal would retire for five minutes to consider the request for further cross-examination. Of course, the only external influence whilst I was under oath, in purdah and giving evidence had come from the Trust team itself, reminding me of the threat of costs. However, the confidence, body language and the gleam in the eyes of the Trust's team suggested that they'd found something very incriminating. I was warned by Paras that if I had indeed been subject to external influences whilst under oath then the whole case might be thrown out leaving me a sitting duck for costs.

Reconvening, Judge Franey requested that I retake the oath and go back under cross-examination.

Conceding that the Daily Mail article seemed culled from my witness statement, the Trust's barrister reopened the cross-examination.

'Mr Duffy, did you speak to a journalist during the breaks and whilst you remained under oath and in purdah?'

'No.'

The questions came think and fast. I thought I was defending my position pretty well, but then came the knockout punch. You could palpably sense the Trust's team leaning forward for a better view of the kill.

'Mr Duffy, would you turn to page 4 of the photocopy of the Daily Mail article in question? You see two paragraphs down? The line about you going home and discussing things with your solicitor?

Can you point to where this line is contained in your witness statement?'

I couldn't, of course.

'So it isn't in your witness statement then? So can you explain to the Panel how this statement from you came to be in the article in question if it is not contained in the witness statement? Is it not indeed the case that you have spoken to a journalist whilst under oath?'

Silence. Everyone's eyes on me.

I explained that I thought that the phrase might have come from an earlier draft of my witness statement.

'So how did this get into the hands of the media?'

I explained that I'd sent copies of the first draft to the GMC, CQC, NHSI, Dep't of Health, NHS England, Public Concern at Work, local MP, the National Guardian's office etc. etc., precisely because I'd been so frightened of underhand legal tactics and gags.

The electric atmosphere collapsed. You could almost palpably feel the collective groan of disbelief from the Trust's team. They really thought they'd cornered me, breaking purdah by talking to a journalist under oath. Even Ameeta Joshi had turned up unexpectedly to watch, despite her cross-examination being terminated early the previous day after we'd been assured that she'd be unavailable the following morning.

The NHS's barrister had built up the tension beautifully, whipping up and baking the perfect dessert of facts and conjecture leading up to the dramatic climax, the flourish and the kill and then *flop*, the whole thing had collapsed into a soggy, sticky mess. It was an expertly laid ambush and I felt so very sorry for him.

Then I reminded myself of how much he was being paid and how much more damage he could have done to my family, my career and my reputation.

The rest of Friday passed with me sitting almost comatose and shaking at the back. I'd come so close to disaster. If the NHS's legal team had convinced the Tribunal that I'd spoken to the press whilst under oath then I'd not only have lost the case but would undoubtedly have had to pay out a totally ruin-some amount of money. I should have been paying attention to Gertie's testimony and completely missed the comment that the extra AAS operating lists at Barrow in Furness were paid at a lesser rate than the rest of the Trust. Luckily, the panel were clearly paying more attention than me and picked up on this but I wondered later how many other things slipped past without me noticing that day.

I crept off back to the train to Lancaster, utterly exhausted and was so shocked and numbed by my experience that I managed to get on the wrong train, hurtling through Lancaster station to my horror. Thankfully, it wasn't non-stop to Glasgow and I managed to get off at Oxenholme in Kendal.

Finally arriving home, I lay down on the bed, still in my pin-stripes and fell into three hours of dreamless, insensible sleep, only waking up when it was fully dark. I don't think that anything has ever come close to the sheer stress and mental trauma of that day and it was as if my brain needed to fully shut down for a few hours to compensate for the previous five days.

Reconvening on Monday morning there were no further traps and the day finished with Paras and the Trust's barrister wrapping up their arguments. Once again, to my astonishment and anger there were implications of fraud on my behalf. We were told that there'd be a written verdict within about four to six weeks.

Retiring back to the claimants' room, Paras seemed confident about the illegal deduction of salary issues and constructive unfair dismissal; less so about the link between these and the whistle-blowing. It all seemed a bit of an anti-climax after the roller-coaster ride of the previous six days. I phoned and thanked Chris, shook hands with Paras and Adam and with gritted teeth, forced myself to shake hands with the NHS's barrister, telling myself that he was just doing his job.

Half an hour later I dazedly climbed back onto the train for Lancaster and home.

CHAPTER SEVEN

The waiting game

I'D BOOKED A FULL TWO WEEKS OFF for the Tribunal in the expectation that we'd be presenting at least half a dozen or so witnesses in support of my pleadings and running my full case. With the dropping out of all my ex-colleagues from Morecambe Bay, the costs threat and the consequent reduction in my evidence, we'd easily finished with four working days to spare. I should have been able to enjoy these precious days at the family home but the week dragged past, seemingly lasting forever. I lay on my bed, trying to get my thoughts and ectopic heart beats back under control. It felt as though I'd gone through the most thorough and horrible violation, as though my own psyche, personality, vocation and self-respect had been repeatedly raped.

I still had no idea how this was going to work out. On top of tearing the family apart, had I now condemned them to suffering a six figure bill? Would the Tribunal believe the Trust's case that I'd invoiced for clinical sessions when I'd not been there, thus implying attempted fraud on my part? How was it possible that they'd carried on using these accusations as evidence even after their own staff had confirmed them to be entirely baseless? If I lost the case based upon those accusations, how would the authorities on the Isle of Man react? Would I find myself unemployed again, unable to support my family and with a £108,000 costs bill to pay? Would the GMC get involved if the Trust had convinced the Tribunal panel that fraud had indeed been attempted? Yes, they probably would. Could I find myself struck off…? Yes, quite possibly. A spell in the slammer for

NHS fraud and forced to pay back the alleged £112,000/year on top of £108,000 costs.........?

I couldn't believe that the NHS had done this to me, yet at the same time was boasting on its 'Freedom to Speak Up' website that:

> We promise that where staff identify a genuine patient safety concern, we shall not treat them with prejudice and they will not suffer any detriment to their career. Instead, we will support them, fully investigate and, if appropriate, act on their concern. We will also give them feedback about how we have responded to the issue they have raised, as soon as possible.

A short while later I found out that the Trust had deleted these promises during the period around the Tribunal hearing.

MY FAMILY, RELATIVES AND FRIENDS were unfailingly supportive but I couldn't seem to snap myself out of a shocked sense of torpor and bewilderment. Until, that is, Dave, one of my old school friends drove up to offer some advice.

David can be blunt and, looking back, some uncompromising, tough advice was exactly what I needed.

'Man up and stop feeling sorry for yourself.' was the essence of Dave's advice, together with a forceful reminder from him of what I'd stood for over the years. 'You should be proud of yourself. You've done the right thing, stood up to a huge organisation. You're still here, they've not broken you. You're not a criminal. You've just done the job that so many other people would have been too frightened to do. So start feeling proud of yourself instead of hiding away and allowing yourself to become a victim.'

It was damn good, sound advice and, delivered forcefully from someone who'd been a trusted friend since I was five years old, it had the desired effect. Heading back to the Isle of Man on the Sunday afternoon, my mood had lightened considerably and I braced myself for the next big event; the written verdict.

CHAPTER EIGHT

Verdict

WE ALL HAVE VIVID MEMORIES of exactly where we were when major, life-changing news comes through. '9-11' and the London tube bombings come to mind as examples.

In this case, I was on the Manannan, the Isle of Man's Steam Packet catamaran on the run-in to Heysham. It was Saturday 9th June, the end of the TT fortnight. The boat smelled of leathers and was packed with bikers.

I was on the outer deck at the stern of the vessel enjoying the fresh air and sunshine and looking forward to seeing my family and possibly even a family roast meal from Fiona when my mobile bleeped as it picked up the English digital reception, presumably from a mast somewhere around Blackpool. It was an email from Chris Thompson, my solicitor from Gateley's. Instantly, my heart was in my mouth.

I knew that the written verdict was imminent and had no idea of what to expect. The Tribunal panel's expressions during the closing arguments had given little away. I opened the text with a dread, heavy heart, wondering if I ought to be closer to the catamaran's bathroom in case I was ill.

I needn't have worried. The Tribunal had unanimously accepted that I was a genuine whistle-blower and I'd also won unanimously on unfair constructive dismissal and unlawful deduction of pay, lost on the evidential link between detriment, dismissal and whistle-blowing. Paras had warned me that weakening my case to try and head off the costs threat might well cost me the link so this wasn't a massive surprise. The huge relief was that each member of the Panel had indeed believed that my whistle-blowing was genuine and had confirmed that I had been unfairly constructively dismissed and had not believed the NHS's case that I had been invoicing fraudulently.

All the way in to Heysham I simply leaned back against the Manannan's railings, emptied my mind and enjoyed the mosaic of clouds and blue sky, the glitter of the sun on the water and the play of sunshine and wind on my face. I was on the way home to my family and we wouldn't have to re-mortgage or sell our home. It felt like a huge burden had been lifted. Not only had we won on the substantive points, but, equally importantly, the vindictive threat of huge and ruinous personal costs was now dead in the water.

Wasn't it?

CHAPTER NINE

Remedy
Another roasting

THE NEXT STAGE in the litigation process was the Remedy Hearing, which was scheduled for July 29th. Having formed the verdict, the panel then had to meet again for legal argument to take place over whether compensation was due and if so, how much.

Mercifully, this was rather less abusive than the original hearing. The Trust's team seemed subdued and I'd received an informal offer of an out-of-court settlement the previous evening.

I wasn't averse to this, but the amount, coming after I'd already been separated from my family for some eighteen months (and was anticipating a further seven to eight years of exile) was so utterly insulting that I had no hesitation in asking Chris in rather fruity language to *please let the UHMB legal team know that they could stick it…* etc. I suspect that he passed the message on without the four letter words and in more moderate legal language.

Chris and I had prepared the Witness Statement for the Remedies Hearing several weeks earlier. In this kind of an Employment Tribunal scenario you can only claim compensation for actual and direct financial loss, not for psychological injury, stress, ill health, loss of family life and so on. Living as I did on the Isle of Man, the losses would mainly be concentrated around the money that had been illegally withheld from my salary through 2015-16, my loss of earnings whilst unemployed in 2016, the losses whilst I built up my earnings from the job at Noble's to the same after-tax level as that which I'd been earning in Morecambe Bay and finally, the ongoing losses incurred by my accommodation costs on the island and travel back to see the family roughly once a fortnight. Usually, Employment Tribunals don't extrapolate losses very far into the future but I thought that there was little harm in pointing out that I'd be looking at working on the Isle of Man for another seven to eight years. Hence, I worked out my future losses too, adding them to the above total. Even I was shocked by the kind of financial penalty that the family was due to endure as a consequence of the NHS's actions.

Just under £290,000 over the nine to ten year period after my constructive unfair dismissal…

Entirely predictably, Morecambe Bay did some rather radically different calculations, working out that I was owed pretty much zilch.

We met to lock horns again on a Friday morning. It seemed odd, making the same journey back that I'd made during those horrendous days in April. This time I made it there without any trim-checks. The usual procedures were observed and we got down to business.

In this case, the Trust had to accept that I'd been constructively unfairly dismissed (i.e. illegally forced out) and there was little point in them contesting this (although they made little effort to disguise their unhappiness at the verdict). Instead, I was initially cross-examined about the sessions which I'd worked but for which the Trust had refused to pay me. Being pushed about the lack of evidence before the Tribunal to show that the sessions had indeed been worked by myself and freed (or so I thought) from the gagging effects of the costs threat, I felt a great deal more confident speaking my mind. Letting my temper show ever so slightly I told the panel that there should have been at least two or three middle managers (amongst a good many others), giving evidence on my behalf and confirming all the elements of my version of events on this point. I emphasised that their absence was purely a consequence of their fear of retaliation from the NHS.

The Trust's team didn't push this point further. I assumed that they didn't wish discussions to stray into the issue of potential witness intimidation.

Instead, I was then cross-examined on my decision to go to the Isle of Man. Why couldn't I take up a job locally? Carlisle? Blackpool? Preston? If the Trust could make this point stick then all my costs of living and working on Manx soil would be struck out. Of course, if I'd gone for a job within commuting distance of Morecambe Bay it would have only been a matter of time before the witch-hunt caught up with me again; especially with plans going back several years to create one huge urological network across Lancashire and South Cumbria. I'd potentially again find myself working alongside the very people who I believed had started the campaign up against me in the first place.

Going further afield, as helpfully pointed out by Judge Franey, wouldn't have gained me anything over the Isle of Man as I'd still be forced to live away from home. I'd also still be within easy range of BAPIO who I believed had clearly taken sides in the dispute over clinical standards and behaviour and I was very fearful of further allegations.

Retiring after lunch to consider the remedy verdict, the panel reconvened at perhaps 3pm. I'd expected a simple one liner and hopefully a sum of compensation but in fact the panel went through each separate claim and counter claim, one by one. It must have taken around thirty to forty minutes.

I recall winning on pretty much all of my costs with the exception of lost private work. As Judge Franey worked his way through the various elements of the remedies we quickly exceeded the derisory out-of-court offer made the previous evening and it became clear that the Tribunal was going to award significantly more than just token damages. I was well aware that there was an absolute ceiling on the pay-out of around £88,000 and the costs to the NHS started to quickly mount towards this ceiling. We were getting very close and my mental calculations were getting ragged when Judge Franey started to conclude the summing up of the remedies. Paras quickly interjected to point out that the Panel hadn't assessed my costs looking forward another seven to eight years.

After a moment of confusion, the panel asked for a further period to consider this. Returning after only a few minutes, they announced that I'd be awarded costs projected forwards for the full period.

Having reached a sum that was clearly well into six figures, it was now evident that the £88,000 cap would be the limiting factor in damages and, adding in the remaining salary illegally deducted from my earnings, the total came to £102,500.

Remarkably, the sum was agreed, totted up on smartphones and wrapped up in just a few quick minutes, with the Trust's barrister seemingly remarkably calm and accepting of the conclusion, in contrast with the ashen faces of the rest of the NHS's legal team. I quietly commented to Adam as we walked away down the corridor to the claimants' room about just how surreal it seemed, hearing the destruction of your lifetime vocation reduced to pounds and pennies.

Arriving in the claimant's room, Paras broke into a huge grin. I think we'd both had to make a major effort to stay poker-faced for the last few minutes and there was a big, emphatic embrace and man hug, swiftly followed by a second hug and high five with Adam.

We'd carried the day and it seemed high time to retire to the nearest pub for a celebratory round of drinks, phoning Chris along the way with thanks and to let him know of the good news.

With some serious disruption on the railways that night, I was about two hours late getting home. However, there can't have been many passengers that evening who endured the whole extra 120 minutes with an inane grin on their face. I'd have been deliriously happy even if I'd had to walk the whole way! Compared with the potentially ruinous situation just weeks earlier that could have forced us to sell the house, this felt like I'd won the lottery.

It's over, I repeatedly told myself. *It's over:*

Only it wasn't.

CHAPTER TEN

More cost threats

A WEEK LATER I was off with my family to the west coast of Ireland for a fortnight's holiday. Fiona had organised it well before the Tribunal hearings and the laid back, pleasant and family-friendly pace of life in Ireland was just what I needed to start the healing process, try to mentally deal with what had happened and start planning for the future, both for myself and the wider family.

We spent a wonderful and precious two weeks on Ireland's wild Atlantic coast, walking, eating and sightseeing together. After a perfect family fortnight full of laughter, salt, sunshine, sea-spray, showers, windburn and that wonderful hospitality and *craic* that Irish pubs dish out in wholesale quantities, we regretfully headed for Dublin and the ferry home to face reality again. I'd heard nothing from Chris and Paras but was familiar enough with the two of them to know that if there was bad news, they'd hold it back until the holiday was over.

In fact, we returned to doubly bad news. Our affectionate old cat, acquired as a rescue kitten when the boys were tiny had died suddenly. He'd always been there and was as much a part of the family as anyone else. The whole family was distraught. Secondly, Capsticks' solicitors had been in touch on behalf of Morecambe Bay NHS Trust. Despite losing the substantive points on constructive dismissal and illegal deduction of salary, they were now planning to take me back to yet another Tribunal hearing for costs, totalling £48,000.

Their justification for this was that I'd wasted their time by withdrawing some of the pleadings on the opening day of the Tribunal.

But of course I'd been intimidated into this by the NHS's original threat of costs of £108,000! It seemed to me to be little more than a further blatant attempt at bullying and threats. I was astounded that Morecambe Bay and their HR department was prepared to squander a five-figure sum of taxpayers money trying to punish still further their ex-Doctor of the Year and his family, despite their Board's promises of no detriment for any whistle-blower.

Once again there was work and preparation to be done, Paras submitting quite a detailed rebuttal of the NHS's case. After some further discussion we agreed to submit a request for counter costs, outlining some of the irregularities in the NHS's own behaviour.

I thought that we stood a good chance of winning our own counter-application for costs. After all, I'd fully declared all evidence, whether it helped or hindered my case. Nothing in my evidence had been redacted nor had I made remarks to witnesses that could be interpreted as being threatening or intimidatory. No costs threats had been made against the Trust's original defence, nor had there been any actions on my part that might have threatened the homes and families of the NHS managers running the case against me. In my opinion, all these things applied in the opposite direction.

I was quite looking forward to the third hearing and had even offered to be recalled as a witness again. Judge Franey had come across as a worldly-wise, attentive, likeable and generally even-handed judge and I thought it highly unlikely that he and the other panel members would endorse the NHS's behaviour during the case. However, on the eve of the hearing on Thursday the 8th November, disaster struck. A sudden storm hit the Isle of Man with a good number of flights being first delayed and then cancelled, my own being one of them. Frustratingly, it was too late to get the Isle of Man Steam Packet ferry that evening and every single seat out of the Isle of Man was booked for the following morning, presumably by passengers from the earlier cancelled flights. Rebooking on to the first Steam Packet ferry out in the morning, this was also cancelled as a consequence of heavy seas.

I'd have no choice but to miss the hearing.

Thankfully, Paras was sanguine about my absence, having already prepared my case and advised me against appearing again as a witness. If I could send screenshots of my cancelled flight over, he'd present my apologies to the Tribunal.

With the ferry cancelled too, I simply went into work as normal at Noble's Hospital, figuring that I'd probably be more relaxed being in my normal work environment and getting on with things, rather than pacing up and down in my flat, chewing my fingernails and wondering if I was about to be stung for a £48,000 bill.

The message came in from Chris, just after the 3pm urological surgery MDT meeting at Noble's.

No costs in either direction.

Chris's summing up?

'Go home and relax. It's over.'

CHAPTER ELEVEN

Picking up the pieces

AS I WRITE THIS, it is Christmas Eve 2018, 5.15 pm and I'm sitting on a train heading for Blackpool, changing at Preston for trains for Lancaster, having just flown out of Ballasalla Airport, Isle of Man to Manchester with Flybe. I'm planning to text Chris and Paras with more thanks and with Christmas wishes to them and their families. Most importantly, I've got a terribly precious Christmas Day tomorrow with the family before heading back to the Isle of Man on Boxing Day, a 3½ hour journey on the Ben-My-Chree whose lounge is now becoming as familiar as my office at work. I'm very, very happy at the prospect of 24 hours at home with Fiona, Edward, Robert and William, as well as Copper and Rusty (the two tiger-striped rescue centre kittens replacing our old cat). My happiness is enhanced still further at the prospect of one of Fiona's exceptional Christmas roasts. However, I'm mentally and physically exhausted, overweight and desperately out of condition after a roller-coaster year of extreme highs and lows.

I've never known fear as tangible as when I was giving evidence under cross-examination with the threat of a £108,000 bill hanging over me. Nor have I ever known relief like that felt on the stern of the Manannan when I'd (wrongly) thought that the threat of costs was over. Ironically, the Employment Tribunal and legal process, which is supposed to be there to protect abused employees from rogue employers, actually managed to inflict an even greater amount of stress and fear on me than Morecambe Bay's Critical Care Division.

At work, I'm relatively happy. Noble's Hospital is safe, friendly, supportive and functional; for me and for the patients. The quality of service is light years away from some of the errors and neglect that I witnessed first-hand in the urology department of Morecambe Bay. The urology and general surgical teams at Noble's are close-knit and committed and I feel comfortable there, in stark contrast to the hatred and fear that characterised my last few years in the NHS.

I'm much less happy in my spare time on the Isle of Man. Visits home seem far too few and far between. I've tried getting home every weekend for a Saturday night with the family, but it's just too exhausting. Whether I fly or take the ferry seems to make little difference. It's still a stressful, exhausting and unpredictable ten to twelve hour round trip, door to door.

Winter is a particular problem. I enjoy the capricious weather on the Manx wild west coast, but storms regularly cut off all travel to and from the island over the autumn, winter and early spring months.

Evenings and weekends are very, very lonely. Facebook Messenger is a godsend, but it's no substitute for sitting round the television or going out for a walk or a meal with the family. Weekends in particular can seem endless. If I'd wanted to live alone like a lonely hermit, I certainly wouldn't have chosen a life as a married surgeon with a wife and three boys that I miss deeply.

Unlike most people, I long for Monday morning and the end of the weekend so that I can be distracted again by my work.

I told the Tribunal back in August that there was no chance of us tearing the family even further apart by moving some family members to the Isle of Man and leaving others in Lancaster. Similarly, the Tribunal accepted that there was no way back for me into the NHS. After all, they had presided over the repeated neglect and mismanagement of patients, constructively dismissed me, presented evidence that could have got me into terrible trouble with alleged financial impropriety and then threatened and intimidated me with a ruin-some bill over our refusal to drop our legal case. Additionally, I have recently found out that my actions in fighting back against my constructive dismissal will almost certainly have resulted in me being put on a national blacklist by the NHS; a near ubiquitous act of retaliation against any employee having the temerity to publicly challenge the might of the NHS over clinical or corporate governance issues.

Finally, the Tribunal openly acknowledged my fears that I am regarded by some ex-colleagues as *unfinished business.* That will remain the situation and it is clear that I now face a good number of further years separation from family, friends and relatives, despite the verdict in the Tribunal. The settlement of £102,500 was welcome and was the maximum that the Tribunal could award, but doesn't bring my retirement much further forward, especially after tax and barely covers the lost earnings and costs of my eighteen months separation from the family to date.

I'm currently engrossed in trying to find a small flat or house to buy. There seems little point in renting for another seven years or so, when I might as well be paying down a second mortgage.

Somehow, I need to get more time back in Lancaster too. There seem to be a hundred-and-one jobs that need doing at home and which would simply happen without particular effort, were I at home every day. Being home for perhaps one evening per fortnight, I wonder if some of the plans for the family home will ever come to fruition.

The future has never seemed so uncertain all the way back to the early 1980's when I struggled so much to get into and to survive medical school. And now there is an extended family to worry about too.

Would all these awful things, false accusations of fraud and financially devious actions, spurious allegations of bullying, racism and abuse and all of the specious detriments including pay cuts, threatened pay cuts, retrospective pay cuts, demotion etc. have happened anyway if I'd simply stayed silent and continued to work to a standard that won for me the Doctor of the Year award?

I think not.

Looking back through the good times and the bad, the laughter and sadness, the companionship and loneliness, lies and truths, love and hatred, the surgical triumphs and misjudgements, elation and exhaustion, life and death.

I just don't see how I could have done anything differently.

UHMB statement:
RESPONSE TO THE MAIL RE ALLEGATIONS MADE BY FORMER CONSULTANT

Dr David Walker, Medical Director, University Hospitals of Morecambe Bay NHS Foundation Trust (UHMBT), said:

'We are disappointed and saddened that Mr Duffy's contractual dispute with the Trust ended with legal proceedings and that he chose not to work with the Trust to resolve his concerns with us informally.

'It is important to note that all the clinical concerns raised by Mr Duffy were appropriately investigated at the time. We would like to reiterate that the tribunal found there was no evidence to support the claim that Mr Duffy was ill-treated or suffered a detriment for raising his concerns.

'The allegations made by Mr Duffy against the three doctors in support of his salary claim in his Employment Tribunal claim were withdrawn by him at the outset of proceedings and were not tested by the tribunal. The Trust strongly disputed the assertions made by Mr Duffy and had spent considerable time preparing a case which would have robustly disputed these claims.

'We continue to employ the two doctors referred to – who are valued members of the Trust.

'We continue to work hard to ensure that we have a supportive culture for our staff – one where staff are able to raise concerns without any fear, and one where safety – both for our patients and our staff – is paramount, and we are pleased that the extensive judgement in this case has recognised this.'

Author's note. There is no mention in the Tribunal's judgement of a supportive culture for staff. Other aspects of this statement are dealt with in earlier chapters.

POSTSCRIPT

Paradise lost, and for what?

In 2001, William, our third son was born. We purchased a dream house just down the road from the Royal Lancaster Infirmary and I settled into what seemed to be the perfect life with Fiona and our young family. Despite early struggles with wet and dry rot in our Victorian house, we soon came to love it and it proved the perfect place for our family to grow up. It was situated within walking distance of the local schools, Lancaster city centre and the hospital, boasting a gorgeous hillside garden with a big lawn for the boys and our new kitten to play on and views out over Morecambe Bay, Lancaster Castle and the distant Cumbrian mountains. My parents and old school friends were one stop down the motorway, we were surrounded by farming relatives, I was doing the job that I loved and felt a true vocation for and it seemed that life just couldn't get any better. (Part I: Chapter Six)

HOW COULD IT ALL have gone so badly wrong? Did I do anything wrong to deserve this? If not, then what roles did the NHS, the regulators, the politicians and the law play in it all? What can be done to prevent this continuing to happen, not just to NHS whistle-blowers but to responsible and caring individuals throughout society?

If the destruction of my vocation had resulted in a lasting improvement in clinical and behavioural standards in Morecambe Bay then at least there'd be something positive to offset against all the negatives. But, incredibly, even as I type this in 2019, I have become aware that the problems continue. Amongst others, yet another major error has occurred, with a patient misdiagnosed as having a benign kidney lump. After a second opinion and an operation elsewhere, the patient proved to have quite an aggressive kidney cancer. So far I have only heard the patient's point of view. But here we are again, in 2019, with what appears to be yet another mistake, compounded once again by what seems to be a failure of candour and openness, and attempts to avoid discussion and acknowledge-ment of the error, ultimately requiring the patient to have to resort to an external review in order to try and get to the truth.

If this were not bad enough, another possible senior resignation is hanging over the urology department. Once again, the trigger is ongoing issues over bullying, prejudice, personal and professional behaviour and concerns over clinical standards.

There seems no end to this.

The President of one of the Surgical Royal Colleges memorably described my predicament as *an across the board failure by the NHS, the regulators and the law in their duty of care to you and the patients.*

He was right.

The NHS, the regulators and the law

All of these three entities loudly and repeatedly proclaim the importance of safeguarding and speaking out to protect others. But the reality is that when it comes to protecting those who step forward, none are fit for purpose.

Whether it is the NHS, the regulators or the law that is scruti-nised, the huge gulf between the false promises of whistle-blower protection and the grim and ongoing reality of day-to-day whistle-blower retaliation is self-evident. Much needs to be done, and we have come no distance at all from the late 1990's, with the Bristol baby scandal and the treatment of whistle-blower and consultant anaesthetist Steve Bolsin in the NHS, which ultimately resulted in him and his family having to move to Australia.

How can this endless cycle be stopped from happening again and again?

The NHS
All mouth and no trousers.

NHS Trusts and their Human Resources departments, regulators, politicians and patient groups all make it clear that each and every NHS employee has an absolute duty to report and act over episodes of neglect and negligence. Yet, despite the desperate need to encourage staff to speak up about dangerous care, the treatment of those individuals who do indeed risk all by stepping forward to do their duty remains brutal and unforgiving in the extreme. Too often, it is the same individuals and groups who make such a play of the need to speak up and who promise absolute protection to those who do, who then deal out the most vicious retribution, or who hypocritically sit on their hands and refuse to intervene when the inevitable witch-hunt gets under way.

It is difficult to describe the sheer intensity of the hatred that can characterise high profile NHS whistle-blower cases. Numerous lives and families have been destroyed by the ferocious retaliation that has followed expressions of concern within the NHS and the breaking of the unwritten code of National Health Service 'omertà'. Decades of selfless hard work and service count for nothing when a whistle-blower is more committed to safety and quality of care than feels comfortable for their managers and colleagues. In my own case, not content with my constructive dismissal and the breaking up of my family, the NHS was then prepared to continue the witch-hunt all the way into the Employment Tribunal and beyond, deleting their promises of whistle-blower protection from their website whilst even going so far as to allege in a sworn statement the possible wrongful claiming by myself of £112,000 per year.

Had such misleading evidence about me been accepted by the Tribunal, I would have undoubtedly lost the case. As UHMB made clear, the witch-hunt would then have been pursued me into a Costs Hearing with a potentially ruinous £108,000 bill as the consequence. A subsequent striking off for financial malfeasance by the General Medical Council and possibly even criminal investigations with a view to recouping the alleged £112,000 per year and a custodial sentence would have completed my family's total obliteration, as well as sending the clearest of messages to anyone else tempted to speak up from within the organisation. Yet in the midst of this I had done precisely nothing wrong other than perhaps articulating my concerns over failing clinical standards, avoidable deaths, avoidable harm, near misses, cover-ups and the exploitation of overtime work a little too assiduously for the NHS's liking.

HISTORICALLY THE NHS has a truly awful reputation for mistreating and abusing whistle-blowers and their families. It was this reputation for extreme retaliation that led to the Francis Report in 2015. This could and should have dealt ruthlessly with the problem of clinical safety and whistle-blower retaliation in the NHS but increasingly looks like a cop-out and missed opportunity.

Perhaps the biggest change that was brought in post-Francis was the introduction of local 'whistle-blower guardians' for NHS Trusts, together with a non-executive director on each board with responsibility for whistle-blowing. These individuals would come under the umbrella of a National Guardian's Office.

However, the very fact that such appointments are needed at all suggests a colossal, across-the-board failure of governance and standards in the heart of the National Health Service. If NHS Trusts, their executives and senior managers could be relied upon to deal appropriately and truthfully with vital information about dangerous clinical and corporate failings then, of course, there'd be no need for guardians at all. Wouldn't it be better to appoint senior managers and executives who can be trusted to act in the best interests of the patients? Instead, we leave in post those who clearly cannot cope with such responsibility and then try to police them with whistle-blower guardians who possess considerably less power than the individuals who they are tasked with controlling. To make things worse, such guardians are themselves employed by and answerable to the very same NHS organisations and senior executives that they are monitoring and holding to account, suggesting a clear conflict of interests.

Instead there needs to be a comprehensive change within senior management and senior members of the medical and nursing professions in the NHS. All too often, senior clinicians, managers and executives are bent upon self-promotion, advancing their own careers ahead of others by giving the impression of being a 'safe' pair of hands, suppressing dissent and ruthlessly dealing with anything that might represent a threat or poor publicity for themselves, the greater organisation or 'the Minister'. With a whole tier of NHS executives knowing that their survival and promotion depends upon exhibiting the same characteristics of cover-up and carry-on, anyone stepping out of line can expect no mercy.

Such a situation is exacerbated by those in lesser management positions who are primarily in post to support such powerful senior managers. Drawn along behind the careers of senior executives like the tail of a comet are dozens of other managers whose job it is to keep things quiet for their executive bosses; at all costs.

The medical profession is no better at robustly standing up for patient interests in this respect. It is well known within the NHS that doctors and consultants in particular are almost un-sackable. Protected by a powerful union, the British Medical Association and appointed on permanent contracts, the power of consultants is bolstered still further by local networks and often tribalistic groups who, it seems, will instinctively close ranks around any underperforming member. These exclusive groups possess the power to be able to materially influence executive decision-making within the NHS. Even Chief Executives need to tread carefully when dealing with such powerful cabals. All too often, the fear of offending such factions results in the retention of staff who are clearly incapable of dealing with responsibility and of delivering uniformly high standards. If any proof were needed, just look at the Ian Paterson case.

Local whistle-blower guardians can never hope to change this long-standing, toxic and dishonest culture. Things will only improve when senior management (including senior medics) are incentivised and motivated to act to preserve high standards and root out underperforming groups and individuals and can enjoy substantive protection and rewards for doing so. It will only be when instinctively right-thinking and, where necessary, outspoken individuals are recruited into, promoted and protected at <u>all</u> levels of the vast NHS machine and are genuinely both motivated and empowered to support both the patients and each other in speaking out against corruption, wastage, negligence, cover-up and complacency that things can begin to change for the better. Only then can the NHS can start to make inroads into its lamentable record for neglect and avoidable deaths and start deploying its taxpayer-derived finances where they can be best utilised.

Such radical change in middle and senior NHS clinicians and management will never be achieved with the current climate of political apathy and denial. Only a clear, courageous and decisive, top down change in direction and leadership style in Whitehall and Westminster will induce the kind of change that is needed if we are to save thousands more patients from avoidable deaths. Managers need to be encouraged to honestly and openly address failings and should be rewarded for doing so. Those who resort to complacency and cover-up should be removed from post, excluding no one if the NHS is to be returned to the kind of focused, committed organisation that our patients and taxpayers have a right to expect.

On its own however, even this will not succeed. Whilst change is needed at the top, there needs to be equivalent change at the front-line too. Those who have historically and understandably stayed silent about NHS errors over fear of demotion, persecution or redundancy need to be positively encouraged and empowered to speak out without fear. There is no point in threatening such individuals with being 'struck-off' by their regulator if they fail to speak up. Nor will they be sweet-talked into speaking out by fine words but without powerful back-up. Their fear of vindictive senior management and clinical colleagues will always greatly outweigh such honeyed words, false promises and toothless threats.

It is only when proper and definitive action to protect whistle-blowers is taken at the very top of the NHS and when the wake of the NHS juggernaut ceases to be littered with the road-kill of whistle-blower's careers and families that the front-line staff will begin to truly believe that they can speak out freely and expect to be robustly supported by an NHS hierarchy and, critically, the regulatory authorities.

Consistent and robust action is needed. Not more words.

The Regulators
Where were they?

There are a bewildering number of regulatory bodies in healthcare, these bodies employing thousands upon thousands of people. In themselves, they are a significant national employer. However, with the possible exception of the GMC, my own personal experience has shown these organisations to be entirely toothless, more interested in denial and shielding themselves from having to take on extra work than in robustly tackling the kind of failures in care that put hundreds of patients at serious risk every week. The CQC, NHSI, National Guardian's Office, NHS England, Coroner's Office, Department of Health and Social Care and the Office of the Secretary of State for Health were all acutely aware of exactly what was going on in my case. All excelled only in weary disinterest, buck-passing, and inventing reasons to excuse themselves from taking responsibility both for the investigation of clinical concerns in the Morecambe Bay urological surgery department and for the protection of those speaking out.

I am far from the only one to have run up against this regulatory brick wall.

Often developing a cosy and mutually serving relationship with the Trusts and NHS organisations that they are tasked with policing, the regulatory bodies simply don't seem to have the courage to tackle powerful and opaque bodies like NHS Foundation Trusts. My own experience is that, despite repeatedly supplying detailed information and contact numbers of eyewitnesses, such regulators prefer to deal with senior executives in the NHS, expressing satisfaction with the comforting lie that all is well, rather than probing deeper into the uncomfortable truths of the often deeply dysfunctional structures within the NHS. Perhaps afraid of what they might find if they shine a light into the deeper, darker recesses of these organisations, the regulators succeed only in further embedding a culture of tolerance of low standards and complacency.

Breaking up the cosy cabal that exists between the NHS and the regulators would go a long way to enhancing clinical safety within the NHS but in itself will not protect those with the commitment to speak out on behalf of wronged patients.

The GMC, NHSI, Department of Health and Social Care, EHRC, local MP's, NHS England, National Guardian's Office etc. have all repeatedly pointed the finger at the Care Quality Commission as being the appropriate organisation to look into departmental clinical concerns and failures and at the same time defend whistle-blowers like myself against the predations of the NHS. But, quite incredibly, the CQC openly admit on their website that, whilst they actively encourage whistle-blowing, they will not take any steps to defend staff who speak out in confidence to them against subsequent retaliation, no matter how serious or genuine the concerns, or how pitiless or illegal the punishment. It is an astonishing policy which seems almost purpose designed to lure well meaning, committed staff into a trap, where they are 'outed' as a whistle-blower and then left defenceless and at the mercy of ruthless NHS HR departments and executives.

Since not one single national regulator has shown any interest whatsoever in supporting victimised whistle-blowers despite some appalling examples of the illegal treatment of such individuals, it stands to reason that the huge black-hole at the centre of UK whistle-blower protection needs to be filled by a new regulator, able to work alongside the existing structures but fully independent. Such a regulator would need to be endowed with the power, utilising litigation if necessary, to reverse the current abuse and victimisation of whistle-blowers. They would need to be equipped with teeth and the courage to use them, holding to account large organisations and powerful individuals who would target their employees simply for doing their job and discharging their moral and professional duties. The existence of such a powerful regulator would usher in a sea change in attitudes to candour and speaking up, with rogue and complacent management no longer able to routinely target vulnerable whistle-blowers with absolute impunity.

However, such a regulator would need to be supported by statutory powers and powerful new legislation that would enable action to be successfully and swiftly undertaken against rogue employers, whilst being resistant to the dishonest and bullying tactics that undermine the current litigation process.

The Law
Never asking the fundamental question.

The Public Interest Disclosure Act (PIDA) was drawn up in 1999 in the wake of a good number of scandals, including the Bristol heart babies scandal. It was undoubtedly a well-intentioned piece of legislation aimed at encouraging individuals to impart sensitive information in the public interest and designed to protect these individuals from retaliation from those threatened by such candour.

Unfortunately the act has never really achieved its desired purpose. Clever lawyers have found a myriad of ways of circumventing the Act and its intentions. This has developed to the point where the PIDA simply serves to produce yet another layer of cover-ups, obscuring the original disclosures as well as providing the vengeful employer with yet another opportunity to threaten and punish the whistle-blower.

Something new, better and fairer is very urgently required.

It is for Parliament to decide upon the correct structure of an act to replace the PIDA, but it seems clear that current legislation fails whistle-blowers in a number of key areas. Any new legislation should be specifically formulated to avoid repeating these failures, level the playing field and close the existing, well known loopholes that are routinely exploited in present day litigation.

Where employees are victimised or dismissed in association with making protected disclosures or whistle-blowing, the current litigation takes far too long. It took well over 18 months after my constructive unfair dismissal for the case to come to the front of the queue. When whistle-blowers are unfairly dismissed or sacked by a monopoly employer like the NHS, the consequences for whistle-blower and family can be catastrophic. Studies by eminent sociologists and psychologists are littered with horrifying statistics about suicide rates, drug dependency, divorce, alcoholism and psychiatric disorders in persecuted whistle-blowers. I was lucky enough to find a job overseas within six months of my dismissal but, had the Isle of Man not come to my rescue, the consequences for the family could have been ruinous in the extreme.

All the time that the case drags out, the regulatory organisations use the existence of ongoing litigation as an excuse for not getting involved. When the litigation is over and after a delay of eighteen months, the same regulators then use the excuse that the case is now historical and time-expired. Hence, there needs to be a way of fast-tracking such cases through to a swift and decisive conclusion.

As well as the inordinate delays, the current process focuses far too much on the character of the whistle-blower rather than on the original disclosures or attempts to protect the public.

It is the ubiquitous response for the defending organisation to produce a vehement, indignant blanket denial of everything, but then to stake out a legal fall-back position. If it fails to convince the Tribunal that its actions were entirely innocent, it then blames the victimisation, abuse and/or dismissal of the whistle-blower on some aspect of the whistle-blower's employment history unconnected with the disclosures themselves.

Known as 'reason-shopping' amongst NHS Human Resources departments and lawyers, the intention is to focus mercilessly on the character of the whistle-blower and lead the Tribunal away from the disclosures and retaliation and instead towards any other flaw or chink in the whistle-blowers employment record that can be put forward as a 'reason' for their victimisation and/or dismissal.

Anything will do. Employment records and internal emails will be scrutinised in the minutest detail in the hope of uncovering and distorting any kind of employment irregularity that might act as a smoke screen or distract the Tribunal from the truth.

The end result of this tactic is that the tables are not-so-subtly turned and it is the whistle-blower who, despite already often being shorn of their vocation and potentially family, friends, relatives and home then becomes the focus once more of hostile accusations and damage to their reputation, a situation made even worse by the fact that the whistle-blower goes under hostile cross-examination first. If they can be broken, silenced or discredited early on in the process then the game is over. The case can be closed down without the employer ever having to produce a single witness.

In situations with an isolated whistle-blower versus a huge organisation (frequently an NHS one) in full denial and retaliation mode, determined to hunt down any indiscretions or exploitable variables in the claimant's records, the presence of written evidence and independent eye witnesses becomes absolutely vital if the Tribunal is to assess the case fairly.

It is a ubiquitous requirement of UK justice that all evidence be disclosed. Similarly, the importance of all witnesses being able to impart their evidence without undue pressure, intimidation, coercion or adverse influence is widely acknowledged and recognised in Law. However, the legal process seems to have strayed a long way from these laudable principles.

In my own case, I was ordered to disclose absolutely everything, even information that might undermine my case, something that I duly complied with. In the NHS's case, emails were redacted (i.e. destroyed; see Part II, chapter four) and with-held and it was even necessary to hold a preliminary hearing to obtain evidence that we knew to exist and had been repeatedly requesting for nearly eighteen months.

Third party witnesses were treated in the same cavalier fashion. Of the ten or so original witnesses from the urology department, not a single one was left after senior management from the Trust met with the consultants and middle grades a few months prior to the hearing, mentioning the closure or 'dissolving' of the department if the case went badly. As for the most important third party witness of all, he was informed that he'd only be allowed to appear for the NHS and, having refused to sign the witness statement prepared for him and having instead written his own, was then informed that he would not be appearing at all and his (highly relevant) self-written statement and evidence would not be seen by the Tribunal.

These tactics do not leave much independent evidence and in my opinion fundamentally undermine the principles upon which the law should rest.

However, there is one remaining source of evidence and that, of course, is the claimant themselves.

With much of the written and third party witness evidence having been closed down and/or compromised, the claimant is by now a sitting duck for a costs threat. This is another commonly deployed tactic and seems to be a particular favourite of NHS Trusts and their HR departments.

> *Drop the case, stay silent, agree to some form of gag and we'll not pursue you for our legal costs when you lose, as we assure you is about to happen.*

Of course, utilising taxpayers' money, the NHS can accrue huge legal costs with aplomb, knowing that as its legal invoices build up, so does the potency of the inevitable *without prejudice save as to costs* letter; £108,000 in my case.

Such cost threats may be legal (although in my opinion they represent a gross distortion of the original intent of such letters) but they are also, I believe, an example of extreme witness intimidation. Some individuals have dropped cases altogether under the pressure of such a threat (the recent Chris Day case comes to mind). In my case, I was intimidated into significantly weakening my case in an ultimately futile attempt to negate the threat of costs to myself and the family. Although the Trust played the litigation game within the parameters of the law, as a main witness it is difficult in my opinion to imagine a more blatant example of witness intimidation.

Such threats are magnified further by the fact that claimants are unable to respond in kind. Even in the highly unlikely event of such a threat being made by a solitary claimant against the employer, any consequent bill would be easily swallowed up by the organisation or, in the case of the NHS, simply handed on to the taxpayer. The executives driving these corrupt costs threats against the whistle-blower and main witness will never know what it is like to find their own financial future and family home threatened.

Once all of these tactics had been deployed, it was perhaps no surprise in my case that the Tribunal were unable to find direct evidence linking my whistle-blowing with my subsequent constructive dismissal. The Tribunal, probably very well aware of these kinds of tactics, commented on the lack of witnesses and the *evidential lacuna* (blank) at the centre of the case.

The most important question by far was, of course, the one that was never asked.

> *Would all these awful things, false accusations of fraud and financially devious actions, spurious allegations of bullying, racism and abuse and all of the specious detriments including pay cuts, threatened pay cuts, retrospective pay cuts, demotion etc. have happened anyway if I'd simply stayed silent and continued to work to a standard that won for me the Doctor of the Year award?*
> *I think not.* (Part II: Chapter 11)

In summary, a successor to the PIDA needs to be framed with all of these flaws and weaknesses in mind if our general public are to be protected from error and neglect and if those who would come forward on behalf of the public are to be protected from retaliation and revenge.

Tribunal Hearings need to take place to a much speedier timetable, possibly via specialist whistle-blowing Employment Tribunals, tasked with fast-tracking cases where there may be a risk to the general public.

It should be mandatory that such hearings look carefully at the magnitude of the disclosures and the rapid deployment of relevant investigatory bodies should be ordered in the event that the public remains at risk. Stringent rules should ensure that the focus remains on the disclosures, the protection of the public and of the whistle-blower and should prevent the tactic of reason-shopping and attempts to convert the process into a trial of the whistle-blower's character and integrity.

Evidence should be rigorously declared and the appropriate conclusions drawn by the tribunal where there is an unwillingness to disclose, or where evidence is destroyed or suppressed.

There should be severe penalties where attempts are made to influence or prevent third party witnesses from appearing before the Tribunal. Attempts to interfere with or pervert such evidence should result in the Tribunal drawing the appropriate conclusions.

The tactic of cost-threats should be banned forthwith.

NHS departments and HR departments are of course all too well aware of the concept of 'plausible deniability' and career assassination; the workings of employment Tribunals and the legal requirements and weaknesses of the PIDA. In an organisation dominated by bullying, cover-ups and abuse, it is far too easy to arrange an entirely deniable career 'accident' for a whistle-blower, which can then be blamed on poor communication, misunderstandings or junior management shortcomings, whilst sending a very clear message indeed to anyone else who might be inclined to speak out.

Bearing this concept of plausible deniability in mind, the legal requirement that the claimant demonstrate an evidential connection between the protected disclosure (whistle-blowing) and detriment (victimisation or dismissal) should be abandoned. Tribunals should be free to ask the obvious question and to use their common-sense and knowledge of employment standards to decide whether the whistle-blowers overall treatment was in any way connected with or influenced by their original disclosures and whether, had the original disclosures not been made, the detriments and/or dismissal would nevertheless have proceeded anyway.

Looking at the numerous hurdles and traps that await any whistle-blower involved in PIDA litigation, it is perhaps no surprise that a recent Parliamentary debate revealed that only about 3% of whistle-blowers win their case under the PIDA.

Successes against big NHS Trusts are almost unheard of.

———————

THE HISTORY OF the NHS and other healthcare organisations around the world has taught us that without strong leadership, standards and discipline it is all too easy for organisations to lapse into apathy, low standards, abuse and cover-ups. Front line staff look the other way and concentrate on keeping their jobs and career prospects, persuading themselves that they will be of more use remaining within a failing service rather than speaking up and being dismissed.

Managers, forever incentivised to cut costs and balance budgets, convince themselves that standards are adequate. *After all, no-one is protesting are they?* Senior executives barely ever venture out of their plush offices and high-powered meetings, contenting themselves with a constant *twitter* commentary on how well they and their organisation are doing.

Overstretched regulators prefer to look the other way rather than take on yet more investigative work. After all, why pursue a demanding and uncomfortable truth when there's always a soothing, comforting, no-effort lie offered as a tempting alternative?

The law rightly proclaims both the core importance of evidence and *equality of arms*, so that lone individuals can, in theory at least, defend themselves against the predations of multi-billion pound organisations. Yet, as it currently operates, the law also permits the destruction and with-holding of evidence, cost-threats and witness intimidation. In this unequal struggle between ant and elephant, the elephant can bend the rules with impunity.

Top politicians and ministers continue to promise and proclaim their loyalty and commitment to whistle-blowers. Such pledges reach a frenzied climax in the aftermath of each health or social care scandal. Yet within days they and their civil servants are refusing any contact with dismissed and targeted whistle blowers.

Laissez-faire; look the other way; cover-up and carry-on. It is all-too-seductive a philosophy when careers and livelihoods may be at stake, including your own.

Until you recall the 11,000 avoidable deaths that continue, every year, right under the gaze of our healthcare system, politicians and regulators.

The case for greatly enhanced organisational, regulatory, legal and political protection for those who would speak up for the greater good is surely beyond contention. There can surely be no alternative if we are to encourage acts of candour and care and protect the most vulnerable in our population from the ongoing and sometimes fatal consequences of complacency and cover-up.

Epilogue

'WHISTLE IN THE WIND' started with a list of NHS failings going back through some 20 years of scandals, errors and avoidable deaths. However, it is important to recognise that such errors and wholesale loss of human life are not exclusive to our own much loved but deeply flawed health service.

The Clapham rail crash, Grenfell, Zebrugge and the Herald of Free Enterprise, the Marchioness disaster, Aberfan, Piper Alpha, to name but a few show that even in modern society we are still deeply afraid of speaking out, declaring concerns and being targeted for doing so, even when we **know** that the lives of our fellow citizens are at stake.

I hope that the reader will be both angered and motivated by my account and will pass on their thoughts and recommend this manuscript to friends and family. I hope their sense of injustice will be enhanced by the thought of the hundreds, probably thousands of NHS whistle-blowers and their families who have suffered similar treatment over the decades. I hope that the reader's emotions will be heightened still further by the thought of the thousands of patients who suffer avoidable death, serious harm or near misses every month in the NHS, with front-line staff too afraid to speak out or safeguard for fear of detriment or dismissal. I hope that readers will be sufficiently motivated to take up these issues with their local MPs, the Department of Health and Social Care, Matt Hancock; the Secretary of State for Health and Social Care; NHS England and so-on.

If my account in some small way helps to inform the debate over safety standards, whistle-blowing, safeguarding and the protection of the general public in both our precious National Health Service

243

and society as a whole, then the ongoing pain and cost to myself and my family may just have been worth it.

Peter Duffy
Peel
Isle of Man
July 2019